Unlocking Social Drivers of Health (SDOH) and Health Equity in Radiology and Imaging

A Stanford Health Care Operations Guide

CONTENTS

ACKNOWLEDGEMENTS iv

FOREWORD 6

SECTION 1: INTRODUCTION AND UNLOCKING HEALTH EQUITY 8

    Stanford Health Care (SHC) Radiology Resource on Social Drivers of Health (SDOH) and Advancing Health Equity 9

    Unlocking Health Equity: Understanding SDOH and Its Role in Healthcare 10

    Key Definitions for Advancing Health Equity in Radiology 12

    Overview of Radiology and Imaging Services at Stanford Medicine 16

    Why It Matters: The Role of SDOH and Health Equity in Radiology 18

    Four (4) Key Takeaways 22

SECTION 2: HISTORICAL CONTEXT OF HEALTH DISPARITIES IN RADIOLOGY 24

    Historical Context of Health Disparities in Radiology 25

    Historical Inequities in Access to Imaging Services for LGBTQIA+ Patients 31

Specific Social Drivers of Health (SDOH) Relevant to Radiology at Stanford 35

Key Milestones and Changes in Radiology 45

Health Equity in Radiology and Imaging at Stanford Medicine 49

Stanford Radiology Demographics and Data 50

Stanford Medicine's Frameworks and Models for Promoting Health Equity 58

Four (4) Key Takeaways 67

SECTION 3: CASE STUDIES ADDRESSING SOCIAL AND COMMUNITY CONTEXT IN RADIOLOGY 69

1. Case Study 1: Social and Community Context 70
2. Case Study 2: Economic Stability in Radiology ... 77
3. Case Study 3: Addressing Education Access and Quality in Radiology 88
4. Case Study 4: Addressing Food Insecurity and Health in Diagnostic Imaging 97
5. Case Study 5: Neighborhood and Built/Physical Environment 106
6. Case Study 6: Addressing Healthcare Access and Quality for Susan Taylor 114

7. Case Study 7: Addressing Sex and Gender Discrimination in Healthcare 121

Four (4) Key Takeaways 129

SECTION 4: TECHNOLOGICAL INNOVATIONS AND HEALTH EQUITY AT STANFORD MEDICINE 131

Technological Innovations and Health Equity at Stanford Medicine 132

Four (4) Key Takeaway 139

SECTION 5: INFLUENCE OF ACADEMIC MEDICAL CENTERS IN ADVANCING HEALTH EQUITY 141

Influence of Academic Medical Centers 142

Four (4) Key Takeaway 149

REFERENCES 151

ACKNOWLEDGEMENTS

The creation of the "Stanford Health Care Radiology Social Determinants of Health (SDOH) Guide" has been a deeply rewarding and transformative project. This comprehensive guide aims to empower radiology professionals by enhancing their understanding of social determinants of health and encouraging the integration of SDOH principles into clinical practice to promote health equity.

I would like to express my sincere gratitude to the core contributors who generously devoted their time, expertise, and support to bring this invaluable resource to fruition. Their profound insights and unwavering commitment were invaluable in shaping this comprehensive guide.

Editors and Main Contributors:

Rachel-Gifty Stewart, MHA
Lead Writer and Editor
Graduate Administrative Intern, Stanford Health Care Radiology Department

Rachel Smith, MS
Senior Program Manager, Strategy and Operations—Imaging Services

Elizabeth Oyekan, PharmD, FCSHP, CPIIQ
VP Pharmacy & Imaging Services, Stanford Health Care (SHC)
Chief Pharmacy Officer, SHC & SHC Tri-Valley

Amy Bui, MPH
Sr. Clinical Data Analyst – Imaging Services

Erin Grady, MD, CCD, FACNM, FSNMMI (she/her)
Associate Chair of Education and Diversity, Equity & Inclusion
Clinical Professor, Stanford Department of Radiology
Nuclear Medicine & Molecular Imaging

Stanford Health Care Contributors:

Sheila Galuppo – Imaging Services Marketing Manager
Kaitlyn McGrath – Director, Program Management, Cancer DSL
Tom Cartwright – Strategy and Operations Leader—Imaging Services

This guide would not have been possible without the dedication and collaborative efforts of this incredible team. Thank you all for your contributions and for advancing our shared mission to address health disparities and ensure equitable access to radiological services.

FOREWORD

As physicians, we take an oath to "do no harm." This profound commitment extends beyond the treatment of disease to understanding the broader influences that can shape a patient's health. In today's world, it is not enough to simply address the physical ailments; we must also consider the *social determinants of health*—those forces that intersect with healthcare and often perpetuate harm if left unaddressed. These factors, rooted in socioeconomic status, race, gender, and access to resources, create barriers to equitable care. They are not theoretical; rather, they yield concrete and discernible impacts on patient outcomes.

Understanding the historical context of these social drivers of health is critical. Many of the challenges patients face today are the result of systemic inequalities that have existed for decades. It is incumbent upon us, as healthcare providers, not only to acknowledge these disparities but also to actively strive towards their eradication. This guide is not a political document—it is an ethical one. It adheres to the core principles of medical ethics:

- Respect for autonomy – Every patient has the right to make informed choices about their healthcare.
- Beneficence – Our duty is to act in the best interests of our patients, ensuring that we provide care that promotes their well-being.

- Non-maleficence – Above all, we must do no harm. This means understanding and mitigating both medical and social factors that could negatively affect our patients.

- Justice – We must provide care that is fair and equitable, ensuring that no patient is disadvantaged by circumstances beyond their control.

In this era of rapidly advancing medical technologies, such as AI and personalized medicine, we have a unique opportunity—and responsibility—to ensure that innovation does not deepen existing disparities. Instead, we must harness these tools to close gaps in care and improve health outcomes for all.

As you read this guide, I encourage you to approach the information with an open mind, embracing a *growth mindset*. Incorporate these insights into your practice, allowing them to inform not just how you treat diseases, but how you care for the *whole person*. Together, we can ensure that our efforts truly serve the best interests of every patient, regardless of their background or circumstances.

Erin Grady, MD, CCD, FACNM, FSNMMI (she/her)
Associate Chair of Education and Diversity, Equity & Inclusion Acting Director of Stanford Theragnostic.
Clinical Professor, Stanford Department of Radiology Nuclear Medicine and Molecular Imaging.

SECTION 1

INTRODUCTION AND UNLOCKING HEALTH EQUITY

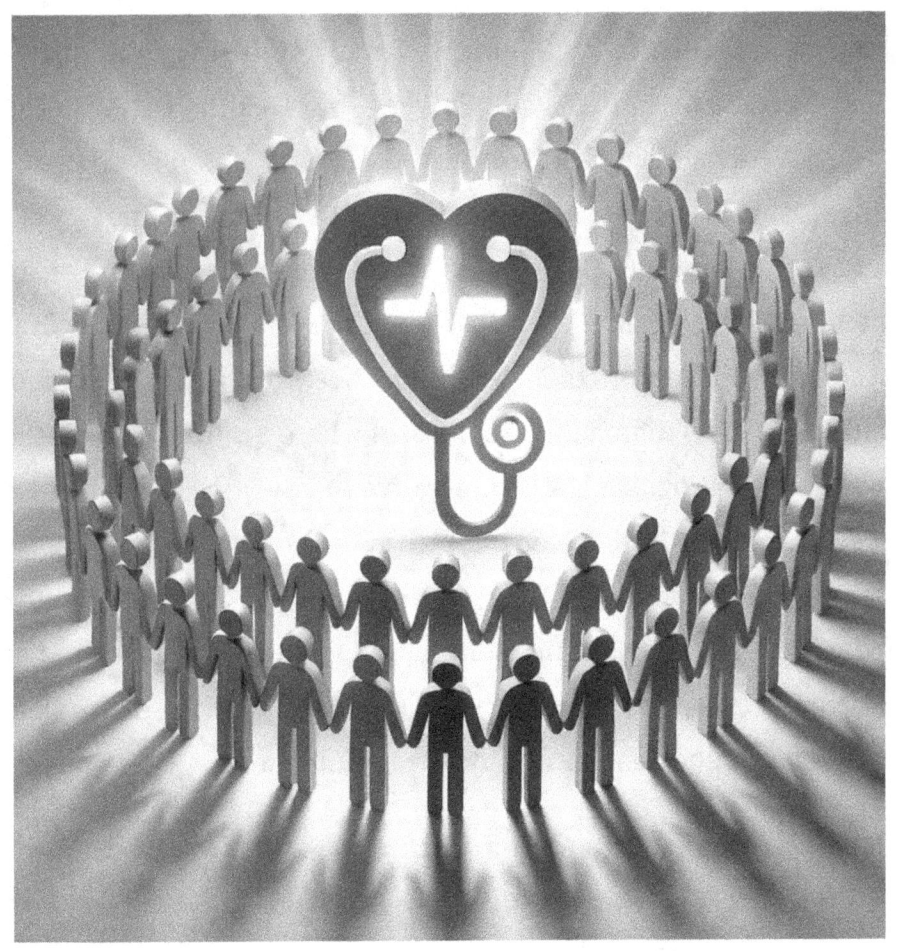

Stanford Health Care (SHC) Radiology Resource on Social Drivers of Health (SDOH) and Advancing Health Equity

Introduction

The **Stanford Health Care Radiology Resource Guide** on Social Drivers of Health (SDOH) and Advancing Health Equity is a critical tool designed to address and mitigate health disparities within radiology. By focusing on how SDOH impacts radiological services and health outcomes, this guide seeks to enhance healthcare providers' awareness and equip them with practical strategies to promote equitable access to imaging. In a world where health disparities are increasingly recognized, it is imperative that healthcare institutions like SHC take proactive steps to bridge the equity gap in radiology. This resource embodies the commitment to diversity, equity, inclusion, and social justice, ultimately striving to ensure that all patients, regardless of their background, receive high-quality imaging care and achieve optimal health outcomes.

"Health equity is the principle underlying a commitment to reduce and ultimately eliminate health disparities that are systematic, avoidable, and unfair."

— Camara Jones

Unlocking Health Equity: Understanding SDOH and Its Role in Healthcare

The concept of health equity is intertwined with the **Social Drivers of Health (SDOH)**—the conditions in which people are born, grow, live, work, and age. SDOH shape the health outcomes of individuals and communities, influencing access to care, quality of treatment, and overall well-being. Factors like neighborhood safety, availability of nutritious food, educational opportunities, and economic stability all contribute to a person's health journey. Acknowledging these factors is fundamental to creating an equitable healthcare system.

Imagine health as a race where some participants must navigate hurdles, while others have a clear path. Health equity is about removing those hurdles—such as limited access to imaging or financial barriers—to ensure that everyone has an equal chance to achieve optimal health. In radiology, this means ensuring that all patients, regardless of socioeconomic background, receive timely and quality imaging services that can lead to early detection and improved treatment outcomes.

The Role of SDOH in Healthcare

SDOH affects every aspect of healthcare delivery and outcomes. They determine who has access to cutting-edge radiology technology, who can afford necessary diagnostic procedures, and who benefits from timely intervention. Achieving health equity requires us to address these underlying drivers to ensure that marginalized populations do not face disproportionate health burdens.

The six key areas of SDOH are:

1. **Food Security**
2. **Healthcare Access and Quality**
3. **Educational Access and Quality**
4. **Physical Environment and Neighborhood**
5. **Social and Community Context**
6. **Economic Stability**

While some refer to SDOH as "determinants," the term **"drivers"** reflects a more dynamic approach, implying that these factors can be influenced and improved through targeted interventions. This guide uses both terms interchangeably but leans towards the concept of "drivers" to reinforce the idea that healthcare providers can take action to mitigate their impact.

Key Definitions for Advancing Health Equity in Radiology

1. Cultural Competency

Definition: The ability of healthcare providers to understand, respect, and effectively interact with patients from diverse backgrounds.

Relation to Radiology: In radiology, cultural competency ensures that patients from various cultural backgrounds receive equitable care. For example, understanding how cultural beliefs might affect a patient's willingness to undergo certain imaging procedures is key to delivering patient-centered care.

2. Cultural Humility

Definition: The practice of self-reflection and awareness of one's own biases while being open to learning from and about others.

Relation to Radiology: By embracing cultural humility, radiologists can build stronger relationships with patients, which leads to more trust and better health outcomes. For instance, a radiologist may need to be open to discussing a patient's cultural apprehensions about certain imaging technologies, which can improve care quality.

3. Race

Definition: A socially constructed category based on physical traits such as skin color.

Relation to Radiology: Understanding how race intersects with healthcare disparities is critical in radiology. Research has shown that minority groups often face delayed diagnosis or misdiagnosis due to implicit biases in imaging interpretation. Combatting these biases can lead to improved care for all racial groups.

4. Social Justice

Definition: The fair distribution of resources, rights, and opportunities within society.

Relation to Radiology: Radiology professionals can advance social justice by advocating for equitable access to imaging services, ensuring that marginalized communities are not left behind when it comes to critical diagnostic tools.

5. Health Equity

Definition: The principle that all individuals should have a fair and just opportunity to attain their highest level of health.

Relation to Radiology: In practice, this means that no patient should experience delays or denials in imaging services based on social factors like income or zip code. Health equity initiatives within radiology departments can include outreach programs to underserved areas and ensure that cutting-edge technologies are accessible to all patients.

6. Implicit Bias

Definition: Unconscious attitudes or stereotypes that affect decisions and actions.

Relation to Radiology: Radiologists must be aware of how implicit biases may influence their diagnosis and treatment decisions. Addressing implicit bias through training and reflection is essential for equitable care.

7. Anti-Racism

Definition: The practice of actively opposing racism and promoting racial equality.

Relation to Radiology: An anti-racist approach in radiology involves confronting disparities in access to diagnostic tools and ensuring that all racial groups are treated fairly in both diagnosis and treatment.

8. Systemic Racism

Definition: Institutionalized policies and practices that create and maintain racial inequalities.

Relation to Radiology: Systemic racism can manifest in limited access to advanced imaging technologies for certain racial or ethnic groups. Radiology professionals can help dismantle these barriers by pushing for policy changes and creating pathways for all patients to access high-quality care.

9. Inequality

Definition: The unequal distribution of resources, treatment, and outcomes.

Relation to Radiology: Radiology professionals can play a pivotal role in addressing healthcare inequalities by ensuring equitable access to diagnostic imaging for all patients, especially those from marginalized communities.

10. Diversity

Definition: The presence of a wide range of different characteristics and identities within a group.

Relation to Radiology: Promoting diversity within radiology teams ensures that healthcare providers reflect the communities they serve, leading to better patient understanding and outcomes.

11. Inclusion

Definition: Actively including diverse individuals and groups in decision-making processes and opportunities.

Relation to Radiology: By fostering an inclusive culture, radiology departments can ensure that every patient feels respected and valued, which can lead to more positive health outcomes.

12. JEDI (Justice, Equity, Diversity, and Inclusion)

Definition: Core principles that promote fairness and respect for all individuals and communities.

Relation to Radiology: Implementing JEDI principles within radiology enhances patient care and creates a workplace where healthcare providers from all backgrounds feel supported.

13. LGBTQ+

Definition: A community that includes individuals with diverse sexual orientations and gender identities.

Relation to Radiology: Radiologists must be aware of the unique health needs of LGBTQ+ patients and ensure that imaging services are delivered in a respectful, affirming, and inclusive manner.

Overview of Radiology and Imaging Services at Stanford Medicine

Stanford Health Care Radiology is a leader in medical imaging, dedicated to delivering exceptional patient care through cutting-edge technology and the expertise of its world-renowned radiologists, technologists, and support staff. The department combines innovation with compassionate care, ensuring that every patient receives the highest standard of diagnostic imaging services. By leveraging the specialized knowledge of Stanford Medicine's distinguished radiologists, the department remains at the forefront of medical advancement, offering services that not only diagnose but also contribute to life-saving treatments.

Stanford Health Care's Radiology and Imaging services encompass a wide range of advanced diagnostic procedures that help detect, diagnose, and treat a variety of medical conditions. From common imaging tests like X-rays and ultrasounds to more complex modalities such as MRI, CT scans, PET scans, and nuclear medicine, the department uses state-of-the-art technology to provide detailed images of the body's internal structures. These images enable healthcare providers to make precise diagnoses and tailor personalized treatment plans, ensuring that every patient receives care that is both effective and individualized.

At the heart of Stanford Radiology's mission is its commitment to three core principles: **care, education, and discovery**. This means not only providing excellent patient care but also fostering a culture of continuous learning and innovation. The department is deeply committed to training the next generation of radiology professionals, advancing the science of imaging, and discovering new techniques and technologies that improve patient outcomes. Every member of the Stanford Radiology team is driven by the shared goal of pushing the boundaries of what is possible in medical imaging, while maintaining the highest level of integrity, empathy, and respect for patients.

The services offered by Stanford Radiology are diverse, spanning diagnostic imaging, interventional radiology, and image-guided therapies. In addition to X-rays, CT scans, MRI, ultrasound, PET scans, and nuclear medicine, the department also excels in **interventional radiology**, a subspecialty that uses imaging to guide minimally invasive procedures for the diagnosis and treatment of diseases. These procedures, which often involve tiny incisions and targeted treatments, provide patients with safer, faster alternatives to traditional surgery. Whether diagnosing cancer, heart disease, or neurological disorders, Stanford's Radiology and Imaging team is focused on delivering precise, timely, and compassionate care.

Why It Matters: The Role of SDOH and Health Equity in Radiology

In the context of radiology, addressing **Social Drivers of Health (SDOH)** and advancing **health equity** are crucial to ensuring that all patients, regardless of their background, have equal access to diagnostic imaging services. The importance of integrating health equity into radiology cannot be overstated, as timely and accurate imaging plays a central role in diagnosing conditions, guiding treatments, and improving overall patient outcomes.

1. **Enhanced Diagnostic Accuracy**: By addressing SDOH—such as transportation difficulties, financial constraints, or

access to healthcare—radiology departments can help ensure that patients receive timely imaging. When imaging services are delayed or missed due to social barriers, the accuracy of diagnoses can suffer. Removing these obstacles improves diagnostic precision and ultimately leads to better patient outcomes. As diagnostic imaging often serves as the first step in a patient's care journey, ensuring timely access can save lives by enabling early detection and treatment.

2. **Improved Access to Imaging Services**: Health equity efforts help bridge the gap between patients who have access to radiology services and those who face barriers due to socioeconomic factors. By understanding the specific challenges patients face, such as lack of transportation or inability to afford services, radiologists and healthcare providers can implement solutions that improve access. This could involve offering flexible scheduling, telehealth consultations, or transportation assistance, ensuring that no patient is deprived of essential diagnostic imaging.

3. **Enhanced Chronic Disease Monitoring**: For patients with chronic conditions such as diabetes, heart disease, or cancer, regular imaging is vital for monitoring disease progression and adjusting treatment plans. Effective SDOH strategies ensure that these patients have consistent access to imaging services, leading to better long-term management of their conditions. Radiologists play a key role in tracking the

health status of these patients over time, providing the data necessary to make informed decisions about their care.

4. **Community Health Impact**: Addressing SDOH within radiology does not just benefit individual patients; it has a ripple effect on the broader community. By ensuring that all community members have access to imaging services, radiology professionals contribute to early disease detection and intervention, which reduces the overall burden of disease in the community. For example, when underserved populations receive timely cancer screenings or cardiovascular imaging, the chances of catching diseases at earlier, more treatable stages increase, improving survival rates and reducing healthcare costs.

5. **Optimal Utilization of Radiology Resources**: Addressing social barriers can also help radiology departments optimize their resources. When patients are unable to attend appointments due to transportation issues or financial hardship, radiology schedules become inefficient, leading to wasted time and resources. By identifying and mitigating these barriers, radiology departments can ensure that their imaging equipment and personnel are used more effectively, reducing no-show rates and improving the flow of patients through the system.

6. **Higher Patient Satisfaction**: Patients who experience fewer barriers to care and are treated with compassion, respect, and cultural sensitivity are more likely to report higher levels of satisfaction with their healthcare experience. When patients feel seen, heard, and supported—whether through empathetic communication or efforts to address their unique challenges—they are more likely to engage in their care and follow through with recommended treatments. Radiology professionals who are mindful of SDOH and health equity are better equipped to create a positive, supportive environment that enhances the overall patient experience.

Stanford Health Care Radiology is not only dedicated to clinical excellence but also to promoting health equity and addressing the social drivers that impact patient access to care. By integrating these principles into its operations, Stanford Radiology ensures that every patient receives timely, accurate, and compassionate imaging services, regardless of their social or economic background. The department's ongoing commitment to innovation, education, and patient-centered care sets a new standard for how radiology can contribute to a more just and equitable healthcare system.

Four (4) Key Takeaways

1. **Health Equity Requires Addressing Social Drivers of Health (SDOH)**: Achieving health equity in radiology demands a deep understanding of the Social Drivers of Health (SDOH), such as food security, access to healthcare, and economic stability. These drivers significantly influence patient outcomes and determine who can access timely and accurate imaging services. Radiology departments must actively address these barriers to ensure equitable care for all patients, regardless of their social circumstances.

2. **The Transition from "Determinants" to "Drivers" Shifts the Paradigm**: The linguistic shift from "Social Determinants" to "Social Drivers" reflects a more dynamic approach to healthcare equity. It emphasizes that while social factors influence health, they are also modifiable through intentional action. This guide embraces the concept of "drivers," highlighting the role healthcare providers can play in mitigating the impacts of these social barriers and improving patient outcomes in radiology.

3. **Cultural Competency and Humility are Central to Equitable Radiology**: Radiology professionals must possess both cultural competency and humility to provide patient-centered care. Cultural competency ensures that radiologists understand and respect patients' diverse backgrounds, while

cultural humility encourages ongoing self-reflection and openness to learning from patients' unique experiences. Together, these principles help radiologists build trust and deliver better health outcomes, especially for underserved communities.

4. **Radiology's Role in Promoting Social Justice and Health Equity**: Radiology departments can play a transformative role in advancing social justice by ensuring equitable access to imaging services. Whether through addressing implicit bias, confronting systemic racism, or advocating for policies that dismantle barriers to care, radiology professionals are uniquely positioned to contribute to a more just healthcare system. By fostering diversity, equity, and inclusion (DEI) within their operations, radiology teams can help eliminate health disparities and improve the overall patient experience.

SECTION 2

HISTORICAL CONTEXT OF HEALTH DISPARITIES IN RADIOLOGY

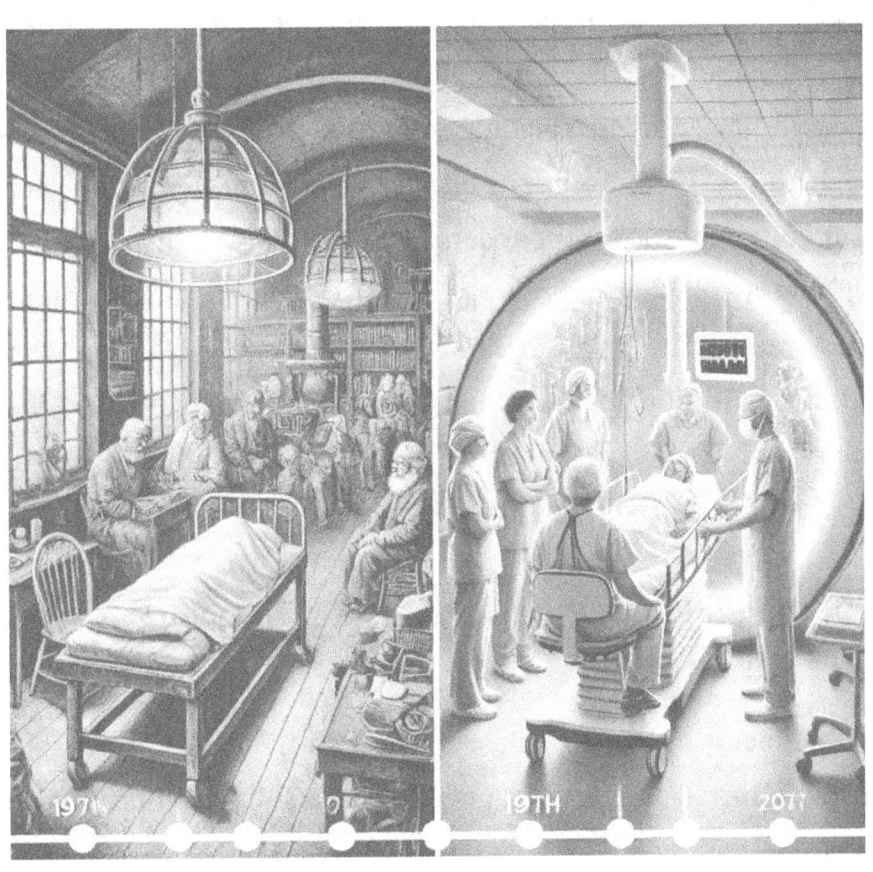

Historical Context of Health Disparities in Radiology

Introduction

For decades, radiology has been both a cornerstone of modern healthcare and a microcosm of its broader inequities. Disparities in access to imaging services mirror long-standing systemic inequities in the healthcare system, with marginalized communities—particularly African Americans—facing disproportionate barriers to care. These disparities are rooted in a complex interplay of factors, including socioeconomic status, race, ethnicity, geography, and entrenched biases within medical institutions. Understanding the historical context of these disparities is crucial to addressing and dismantling them, ensuring that the future of radiology is one of equity and inclusion.

1. *Radiology's Role in Perpetuating Health Disparities*

Radiology professionals, particularly in high-stakes subspecialties like breast imaging, nuclear medicine, interventional radiology, and body imaging, interact with patients across the healthcare continuum, often playing a key role in early diagnosis and treatment. However, despite its critical importance, radiology has historically been a vehicle for the perpetuation of health disparities. From unequal access to imaging technology to the underrepresentation of minority radiologists, the field reflects the broader social inequities that have plagued healthcare for generations.

2. Historical Inequities in Access to Imaging Services for African Americans

The historical exclusion of African Americans from equal access to radiology services is a stark example of how institutional racism has been woven into the fabric of medical practice. According to the **Radiological Society of North America (RSNA)**, both the underrepresentation of Black physicians in radiology and the persistent gaps in access to diagnostic imaging for Black patients are contemporary manifestations of deeply ingrained anti-Black prejudice in healthcare.

From the early 20th century, as radiology developed into a clinical specialty, institutional policies systematically discriminated against Black patients and professionals. Medical associations at the time endorsed discriminatory practices, constructing formidable barriers to the participation of Black radiologists and limiting their ability to influence the field. Black patients, meanwhile, were often denied access to the same diagnostic technologies and treatments available to white patients, contributing to poorer health outcomes.

One of the most egregious examples of this occurred on **May 23, 1968**, when Howard Goldman, Director of the New York Bureau of X-Ray Technology, revealed in Senate hearings that Black patients were routinely given higher radiation doses than white patients. X-ray technicians were instructed by manufacturers to adjust radiation doses based on racist assumptions that Black patients had "harder bones" or "denser skin." A 1968 survey found that 75 out of 90 X-ray technicians in the San Francisco Bay Area admitted to regularly increasing radiation doses for Black patients, with some justifying this practice with pseudoscientific beliefs.

The revelations of these practices prompted public outrage and led to demands for reform from both state and federal authorities. However, the concept of racial adjustment in medical procedures has received little attention in the 21st century, despite growing awareness of the intersection of race and medicine. This history is not just a reflection of past injustices; it underscores the ongoing need to interrogate the use of race in clinical practice and eliminate any lingering biases that may still affect patient care today.

3. *Lessons from History and the Path to Equity*

The misuse of racial categories in radiology, particularly the practice of adjusting radiation doses based on race, highlights how deeply flawed assumptions about biological differences between races have shaped American medical philosophy and practice. These practices were not only harmful to patients but also created a legacy of mistrust and unequal care that continues to affect healthcare delivery. As we engage in contemporary debates over the role of race in medicine, these historical examples remind us of the dangers of using race as a proxy for biological differences and the importance of developing practices that treat patients as individuals, not as representatives of a racial category.

One positive step toward mitigating these inequities came in 1977 when the **International Commission on Radiological Protection (ICRP)** introduced the **"As Low As Reasonably Achievable" (ALARA)** principle, which mandates minimizing radiation exposure for all patients. This was a crucial milestone in creating a more equitable standard of care in radiology. Additionally, advancements like **Automatic Exposure Control (AEC)** have been developed to automatically adjust radiation doses based on patient size and anatomy, ensuring that all patients receive the appropriate dose regardless of race or other characteristics.

4. *Innovation and Progress in Reducing Radiation Exposure*

Today, Stanford Health Care's Department of Radiology builds on this legacy of innovation, pioneering new methods to reduce radiation exposure for all patients. Modern diagnostic imaging technologies, including faster **multi-detector CT scanners**, allow radiologists to capture high-quality images while minimizing radiation doses. These advances not only improve patient safety but also help address disparities in care by ensuring that marginalized populations—who may historically have been exposed to higher radiation levels—receive the same standard of care as others.

One area where Stanford is particularly leading the charge is in the implementation of **cumulative dose tracking measures**. By carefully monitoring the total amount of radiation a patient has been exposed to over time, healthcare providers can further reduce unnecessary radiation exposure, particularly for patients who require frequent imaging due to chronic health conditions. This practice is critical in preventing the harmful long-term effects of radiation and ensuring that vulnerable populations are not disproportionately affected.

Radiation doses are now measured in **millisieverts (mSv)**, with the average annual background radiation exposure ranging from 3 to 5 mSv. In comparison, modern imaging techniques often use far lower doses, making the risk of radiation-related harm negligible. Stanford is also adhering to recommendations from the **National Council on Radiation Protection and Measurements (NCRP)** and the **American Association of Physicists in Medicine (AAPM)** to discontinue the use of **gonadal shielding (GS)** in diagnostic imaging. This change, driven by scientific advancements and a deeper understanding of radiation risks, reflects the institution's commitment to providing evidence-based care that reduces unnecessary interventions while maintaining high standards of safety.

5. A Legacy of Leadership in Radiology Innovation

Stanford Health Care has long been a leader in advancing radiology, not just in terms of technology, but also in the application of ethical and equitable care practices. The institution has pioneered numerous innovations in image-based patient care, research, and education, and its ongoing commitment to reducing radiation dose and improving safety measures is a testament to its leadership in the field.

In conclusion, the historical context of health disparities in radiology serves as a powerful reminder of the work that remains to be done. While significant progress has been made through technological innovation, policy reforms, and increased awareness of the social determinants of health, systemic inequities still persist. By acknowledging the mistakes of the past and continuing to push for equity in all aspects of care, Stanford and other leading institutions have the opportunity to transform radiology into a truly inclusive field where all patients receive the highest standard of care, regardless of their background.

Historical Inequities in Access to Imaging Services for LGBTQIA+ Patients

For many LGBTQIA+ patients, accessing healthcare has long been fraught with barriers, from stigmatization to inadequate medical training on their unique health needs. Radiology, as a critical component of healthcare, is no exception. Historical inequities in access to imaging services for LGBTQIA+ individuals are reflective of broader societal biases, which have shaped the way healthcare is provided to this community. The result is a complex web of health disparities that continues to hinder LGBTQIA+ patients from receiving the compassionate and competent care they deserve.

A Legacy of Discrimination and Stigmatization in Healthcare

LGBTQIA+ individuals often face **systemic discrimination** in healthcare settings. This is particularly evident in radiology, where a lack of understanding about sexual orientation, gender identity, and the specific health risks associated with LGBTQIA+ populations can lead to substandard care. **Stigmatization**—rooted in both societal prejudice and the medical community's historical neglect of LGBTQIA+ health—has contributed to an environment where patients often feel unsafe or unwelcome. For instance, radiology professionals may be unprepared to address the unique screening needs of transgender individuals undergoing hormone therapy or gender-affirming surgeries.

Moreover, **disparities in access to healthcare services**—compounded by lower average incomes and limited access to health insurance—create significant obstacles for LGBTQIA+ patients. Without equitable access to these essential services, members of this community are more likely to experience delayed diagnoses and untreated health conditions, exacerbating already wide health disparities.

Gaps in Medical Education and Training

Despite the recommendations from organizations such as the **Association of American Medical Colleges (AAMC)** and **The Joint Commission** to incorporate LGBTQIA+-specific health education into medical training, there is still a significant gap in the healthcare knowledge of many providers. A study by **Obedin-Maliver et al.** in 2011 revealed that medical students receive, on average, only **five hours of LGBTQIA+-specific training** during their education. Only one-third of courses cover crucial topics such as hormone therapy, surgical transitioning, or cancer screening recommendations for LGBTQIA+ patients.

This lack of training has far-reaching consequences in radiology, where clinicians may feel unprepared or uncomfortable addressing the unique needs of LGBTQIA+ patients. The **absence**

of culturally competent care often leads to substandard healthcare delivery, marked by miscommunication, discomfort, or implicit bias. For example, radiology professionals may fail to understand the necessity of breast cancer screenings for transgender men who have not undergone top surgery, or they may be unaware of the increased risk of certain cancers among transgender women undergoing long-term hormone replacement therapy.

Education and Training: The Path to Equity

Addressing these disparities requires a **comprehensive overhaul of medical education** and training. Healthcare providers, including radiologists and imaging technologists, must be equipped with the knowledge and skills needed to care for LGBTQIA+ patients in a respectful, affirming, and clinically competent manner. This education should include:

1. **Appropriate terminology and communication strategies**: Providers must learn to use the correct pronouns and understand the differences between sexual orientation and gender identity. Establishing respectful communication is essential for building trust with LGBTQIA+ patients.
2. **Gender-affirming surgical procedures and hormone therapy**: Radiology professionals need to understand the imaging requirements associated with gender-affirming

surgeries, such as post-operative imaging for transgender women who have undergone vaginoplasty or breast augmentation, or for transgender men who have had top surgery. Understanding the effects of hormone therapy on the body is also crucial for accurate imaging interpretation.

3. **Mental health and healthcare disparities**: Providers must be trained to recognize the higher prevalence of mental health disorders, substance abuse, and chronic illnesses within the LGBTQIA+ community and how these factors intersect with their imaging needs.

4. **Screening recommendations**: LGBTQIA+ patients often have unique screening needs, such as routine STI or cancer screenings that are tailored to their specific risk factors. Radiologists and imaging technologists must be well-versed in these recommendations to ensure that LGBTQIA+ patients receive the preventive care they need.

5. Training programs should be implemented across all levels of medical education—from undergraduate medical students to practicing clinicians—and continuously updated to reflect evolving terminology, guidelines, and best practices.

Moving Toward an Inclusive Future in Radiology

As the healthcare landscape evolves, radiology departments must be at the forefront of efforts to **eliminate disparities and**

ensure equitable access to imaging services for LGBTQIA+ patients. By fostering an environment of cultural competence, radiology can play a critical role in addressing the health inequities that have long affected this community.

At the institutional level, radiology departments should develop **LGBTQIA+-specific policies and protocols** to ensure that patients receive care that is respectful, affirming, and clinically appropriate. This includes creating safe, welcoming spaces for LGBTQIA+ patients and working to eliminate the barriers that have historically prevented them from accessing quality imaging services.

In doing so, radiology professionals can help build a more equitable healthcare system where every patient, regardless of sexual orientation or gender identity, receives the compassionate and competent care they deserve.

Specific Social Drivers of Health (SDOH) Relevant to Radiology at Stanford

Social Drivers of Health (SDOH) are deeply intertwined with community-level conditions and affect individual health outcomes in profound ways. These social, economic, and environmental factors influence a patient's access to healthcare services, including radiology, and can lead to significant disparities in care. Radiology services at Stanford are not immune to these broader societal inequities, and understanding how SDOH affects patients is crucial for improving access to diagnostic imaging and advancing health equity.

Healthcare systems, such as Stanford, that actively engage with the communities they serve can better address the barriers that prevent individuals from receiving the care they need. By recognizing and addressing SDOH at the community level, healthcare providers can tailor their services to improve patient outcomes and provide more equitable care.

1. Economic Stability

Economic instability is a significant barrier to accessing healthcare, particularly in high-cost regions like Northern California. Approximately **12% of residents** in Northern California live below the poverty line, which directly impacts their ability to access timely imaging services and other essential healthcare.

City's Unemployment Rate Stood at 3.8% in February

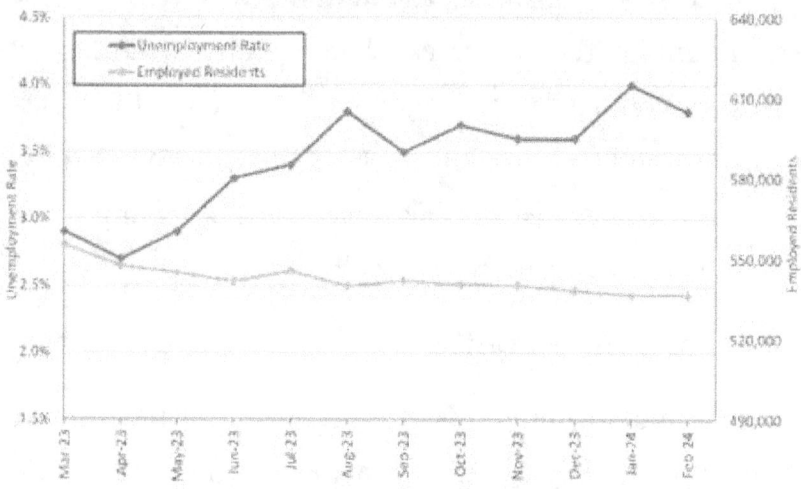

Monthly Unemployment Rate and Employed Residents, San Francisco, Through February 2024

Source: EDD

Recent economic shifts, particularly the loss of tech jobs in the Bay Area, have further exacerbated these disparities. Between 2023 and March 2024, the Bay Area saw a loss of **49,700 tech jobs**, with significant reductions in the San Francisco-San Mateo region. As job losses continue to affect households, many residents are struggling with healthcare affordability, resulting in delayed medical imaging, untreated conditions, and ultimately, worsened health outcomes. Economic downturns can have a cascading effect, where individuals defer preventive imaging or delay seeking diagnostic tests due to financial constraints.

In radiology, economic instability means that patients are less likely to undergo routine screenings such as mammograms, leading to late-stage diagnoses of diseases like breast cancer, which could have been detected earlier with timely imaging. **Stanford Radiology** is committed to mitigating these barriers by offering financial assistance programs and working with community organizations to expand access to imaging for economically disadvantaged patients.

2. Education and Health Literacy

Educational attainment is closely linked to health outcomes. In Northern California, disparities in education levels are stark, with only **24–26%** of Black/African American, Pacific Islander, and Asian residents holding a bachelor's degree or higher, compared to **74%** of White residents. These gaps in education contribute to differences in health literacy, which in turn affect patients' ability to navigate the healthcare system and understand their medical needs.

Health literacy is particularly important in radiology, where patients must understand preparation instructions for imaging procedures, follow-up care, and the implications of their diagnostic results. Low literacy can lead to errors in following treatment plans, increased healthcare costs, and reduced utilization of preventive services like screenings.

For example, patients with limited health literacy may struggle to understand the need for fasting before certain imaging tests or may misinterpret follow-up instructions, which can affect the quality of their care. **Stanford Radiology** addresses this challenge by providing patient education materials that are accessible and easy to understand, ensuring that all patients, regardless of their education level, can make informed decisions about their health.

Red Flags Indicating Limited Health Literacy
• Seeking help only when illness is advanced
• History of missed appointments
• Inaccurate registration forms and other paperwork
• An inability to name their medications or explain why they are taking the medication
• Absence of questions

The **teach-back method** is one strategy used by radiology providers at Stanford to assess and improve patient understanding. This method encourages patients to explain their care instructions in their own words, allowing providers to identify gaps in understanding and clarify information as needed. By fostering clear communication, the teach-back method helps ensure that patients fully grasp their medical needs and are better equipped to manage their health.

3. Social and Community Context

Social and community factors, such as support networks and exposure to discrimination, significantly impact healthcare access and outcomes. Racial and ethnic minorities, in particular, face systemic barriers within healthcare systems that affect their ability to receive timely and high-quality care.

For example, Black individuals in the U.S. are more likely to experience delays in receiving preventive care, which contributes to higher rates of chronic diseases such as hypertension and diabetes. In radiology, this can translate into delayed imaging for conditions that require routine monitoring, such as cardiovascular disease or cancer, leading to poorer health outcomes. **Social isolation**, lack of community support, and fear of discrimination can prevent patients from seeking necessary imaging services.

Women, LGBTQIA+ individuals, and other marginalized groups also experience significant disparities in healthcare access. Women often face challenges in accessing reproductive health services and may encounter bias in pain management or delayed diagnostic services for conditions like endometriosis or fibroids. Similarly, LGBTQIA+ individuals may avoid healthcare settings due to fear of discrimination, further delaying diagnostic tests and preventive screenings that are critical for maintaining health.

Stanford Radiology is actively working to create an inclusive environment that addresses these disparities by fostering a culture of **cultural competence** and engaging with local communities to reduce healthcare barriers. By prioritizing respectful and affirming care for all patients, Stanford is helping to break down the social barriers that have historically limited access to diagnostic imaging.

4. Healthcare Access

Access to healthcare services is a fundamental determinant of health, yet significant disparities persist across the Bay Area. A recent analysis revealed that the percentage of **uninsured Hispanic/Latino individuals** is nearly four times higher than that of White individuals, contributing to unequal access to healthcare and radiology services.

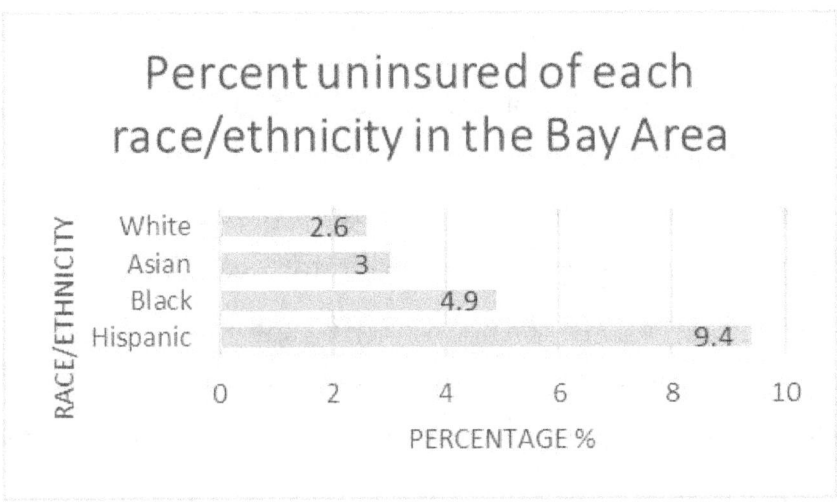

Source: U.S. Census Bureau's ACS 2019 five-year estimates • These figures do not include institutionalized individuals.

Geographic factors also contribute to healthcare access disparities. Urban areas tend to have more extensive healthcare resources, while residents of rural or underserved areas face barriers such as **distance from major medical centers** and **limited transportation options**. In the context of radiology, this can mean that patients in rural areas may have to travel long distances to receive imaging services, leading to delays in diagnosis and treatment.

Stanford Health Care is addressing these geographic disparities by expanding telemedicine and mobile imaging services, ensuring that patients in remote areas can still receive timely diagnostic care. These initiatives are critical for providing equitable access to radiology services, particularly for vulnerable populations.

5. Neighborhood Environment

Environmental factors, such as air quality and housing conditions, have a significant impact on health outcomes. In Northern California, **15% of residents** live in areas with poor air quality, which can exacerbate respiratory conditions and other health concerns. The Bay Area's transportation infrastructure, situated along the bay, is also vulnerable to climate change, with flooding and wildfires posing growing risks to community health.

Neighborhood environments directly affect healthcare access. For example, individuals living in areas with poor infrastructure may face difficulties in reaching healthcare facilities, particularly during extreme weather events. Moreover, low-income neighborhoods often have fewer healthcare resources, leading to increased reliance on emergency services for non-urgent care.

To address these challenges, **Stanford Radiology** is working to provide mobile imaging units and portable diagnostic tools that can be deployed in non-traditional settings. This allows for greater flexibility in delivering care to patients in environmentally vulnerable areas, ensuring that all individuals have access to the imaging services they need.

6. Food Insecurity

Food insecurity is a significant social driver of health that affects more than **1 in 10** residents in the Bay Area. Individuals who experience food insecurity often face a range of health challenges, including higher rates of chronic diseases such as diabetes, hypertension, and heart disease.

The relationship between food insecurity and health is particularly important in radiology, where **nutrition-sensitive conditions** require regular monitoring through imaging. For example, patients with diabetes may need routine imaging to assess complications, such as neuropathy or vascular disease. However, those struggling with food insecurity may prioritize immediate needs, such as securing meals, over preventive healthcare services.

To combat food insecurity, **Stanford Health Care** partners with local food banks and community organizations to address both the immediate needs of vulnerable populations and the long-term health outcomes associated with poor nutrition. By engaging in community-level efforts, Stanford is helping to reduce the broader social drivers that contribute to health disparities.

Addressing **Social Drivers of Health (SDOH)** is crucial for reducing disparities in radiology and ensuring that all patients have access to the imaging services they need. At **Stanford Radiology**, understanding and mitigating the effects of SDOH at the community level is a priority. Through targeted programs, patient education initiatives, and partnerships with local organizations, Stanford is working to close the gaps in healthcare access and improve outcomes for all patients, regardless of their socioeconomic or geographic circumstances.

Key Milestones and Changes in Radiology

Radiology has undergone transformative changes over the years, with innovations that have not only improved patient care but also addressed historical inequities in healthcare. As we advance, it's crucial to reflect on how racial categories and race-based adjustments, even when intended to benefit patients, can sometimes perpetuate biases. Physicians and radiologists must carefully evaluate the evidence, interrogate the underlying assumptions, and consider potential harms when making decisions about diagnosis and treatment. By learning from history, radiology can forge a path forward that prioritizes equity and accuracy.

Dose Modulation and Patient-Specific Imaging

One of the most significant milestones in radiology is the development of **dose modulation** technology, which enables personalized imaging by adjusting the radiation dose based on a patient's body size, shape, and specific anatomical region. This innovation ensures that each patient receives the lowest possible radiation dose necessary to maintain image quality, protecting them from unnecessary exposure while still capturing accurate diagnostic images.

This is particularly critical for **overweight and obese patients**, who may require higher radiation doses to achieve the same image clarity as those with smaller body sizes. With the introduction of **Automatic Exposure Control (AEC)** technology, radiologists can now automatically adjust radiation levels in real-time. AEC systems analyze the patient's tissue density and anatomical characteristics, allowing for more precise imaging and reduced radiation exposure, ensuring that all patients—regardless of body size—receive safe and effective care.

This breakthrough represents a significant shift in radiology, prioritizing patient safety and individualized care. As healthcare becomes more tailored to the unique needs of each individual, dose modulation stands as a vital tool for ensuring that the benefits of imaging are not offset by the risks of overexposure.

Portable and Point-of-Care Imaging: Expanding Access

Another transformative advancement in radiology is the **development of portable and point-of-care imaging devices**. These innovations have expanded access to imaging services, particularly in underserved and remote areas where access to traditional imaging centers may be limited. Portable devices like **Stanford's portable ultrasound systems** offer high-quality imaging in non-traditional healthcare settings, such as rural clinics, emergency rooms, or even home care environments.

The evolution of portable ultrasound technology, which has been progressing for years, now incorporates advanced imaging capabilities, improved portability, and user-friendly designs, making it easier for healthcare providers to deliver care in a variety of settings. These advancements are particularly crucial for **underserved populations** that may face barriers to accessing hospital-based imaging services due to geographic, economic, or mobility constraints.

By bringing imaging to the patient, rather than requiring the patient to travel to a distant facility, portable imaging devices have the potential to **bridge healthcare gaps**, reduce diagnostic delays, and improve patient outcomes—especially for those in rural and low-resource settings. This represents a significant step forward in achieving health equity, as radiology services become more accessible to all populations, regardless of their location or socioeconomic status.

Artificial Intelligence (AI) in Radiology: A New Era of Precision

As radiology continues to evolve, **artificial intelligence (AI)** is playing an increasingly important role in improving diagnostic accuracy and efficiency. AI-powered **decision support tools** are designed to assist radiologists by analyzing complex imaging data, identifying patterns, and providing real-time insights that can enhance clinical decision-making. These tools help reduce human error, ensure consistency in image interpretation, and enable radiologists to detect abnormalities more quickly and accurately.

AI has the potential to significantly reduce healthcare disparities by making advanced diagnostic tools available to a wider range of patients. For example, AI-driven algorithms can assist in screening large populations for conditions like lung cancer or breast cancer, enabling earlier detection and more timely treatment, especially in underserved communities that might otherwise lack access to such cutting-edge technology.

Additionally, AI can help standardize care by reducing the variability that often occurs between different radiologists or imaging centers. By offering consistent, high-quality interpretations, AI tools can enhance the overall quality of care across healthcare systems, ensuring that all patients—regardless of where they receive their imaging—have access to the same level of diagnostic precision.

Looking Forward: The Future of Radiology

These advancements represent just a few of the key milestones that are reshaping the field of radiology. From **dose modulation** and **portable imaging** to the integration of **AI-powered diagnostic tools**, radiology is becoming more patient-centered, accessible, and equitable. However, as we embrace these innovations, it is essential to remain vigilant about potential biases and ensure that new technologies are implemented in a way that benefits all patients.

As AI and other technologies continue to evolve, radiologists will need to remain at the forefront of **ethical decision-making**, ensuring that these tools are used to reduce disparities and improve health outcomes for all populations. With ongoing research and a commitment to innovation, radiology will continue to play a crucial role in advancing healthcare equity, improving patient safety, and transforming the way we diagnose and treat diseases.

Health Equity in Radiology and Imaging at Stanford Medicine

Health equity in radiology and imaging at **Stanford Medicine** is about ensuring that every patient, regardless of race, ethnicity, socioeconomic status, or geographic location, has equal access to high-quality imaging services. The goal is to dismantle healthcare disparities that disproportionately affect marginalized communities and provide patient-centered care that addresses the unique needs of every individual. By promoting diversity, equity, and inclusion (DEI) across all radiology practices, Stanford Medicine works to improve patient outcomes, enhance healthcare delivery, and address social determinants of health that contribute to disparities in diagnostic imaging.

Stanford's commitment to health equity is supported by a variety of initiatives, including **cultural competency training**, **community outreach programs**, and **research on health disparities**. These efforts aim to equip healthcare providers with the tools to better understand and meet the needs of diverse patient populations. The focus is not just on providing imaging services but also on ensuring that every patient feels respected, heard, and valued in the healthcare process.

Stanford Radiology Demographics and Data

According to demographic data from **Stanford Health Care Radiology**, the patient population represents significant diversity in racial and ethnic backgrounds. The hospital serves patients from all over California, with the largest populations coming **Santa Clara County (31.9%)** and **San Mateo County (21.1%)**, and smaller percentages from **Fresno (1.5%)** and **San Francisco (1.8%)**. The wide geographic distribution highlights Stanford's role as a central hub for advanced imaging services, drawing patients from underserved areas as well as major urban centers. Despite this reach, the data also reveal areas where disparities still exist, particularly in access to preventive screenings like breast, prostate, and lung cancer screening.

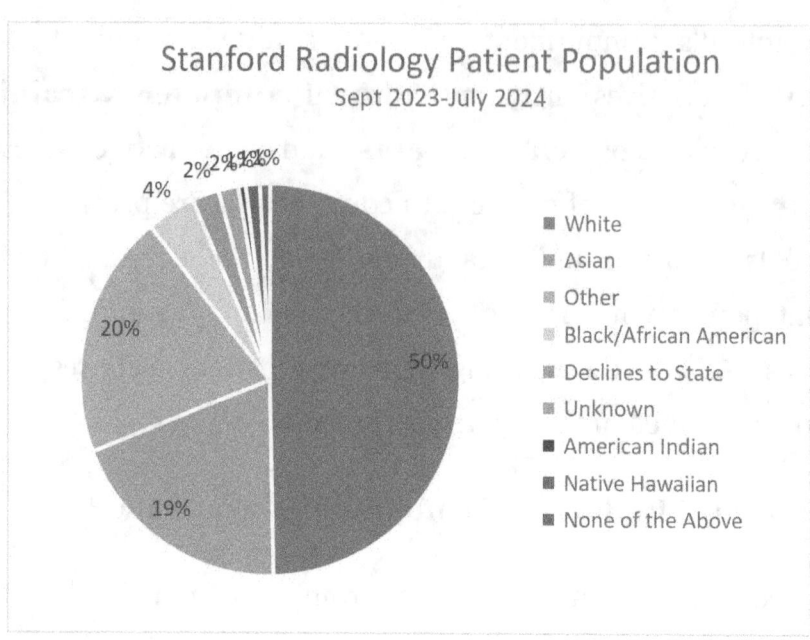

1. Addressing Disparities in Breast Cancer Screening

Data from the **Stanford Cancer Health Equity and Patient Advocacy Committee** and the **Breast Health Equity Subgroup** reveals a significant disparity in breast cancer screening rates for African American women aged 40-49, compared to the general population. While Stanford's overall breast cancer screening rate for patients aged 50-74 is 81%, the rate drops to **50%** for African American women in the 40-49 age group. This gap reflects broader challenges around inconsistent screening guidelines and access to healthcare for younger African

American women, which contributes to later-stage breast cancer diagnoses and poorer outcomes.

To tackle this issue, Stanford conducted **focus group sessions** in the **East Bay region** to better understand the screening practices, risk assessment processes, and barriers faced by African American women. Data from 5,232 women aged 40-49 with recent primary care visits revealed disparities in mammogram order rates across racial and ethnic groups, underscoring the need for targeted interventions. These efforts include increasing patient and provider awareness about early screening recommendations, removing financial and logistical barriers, and improving access to imaging services for at-risk populations.

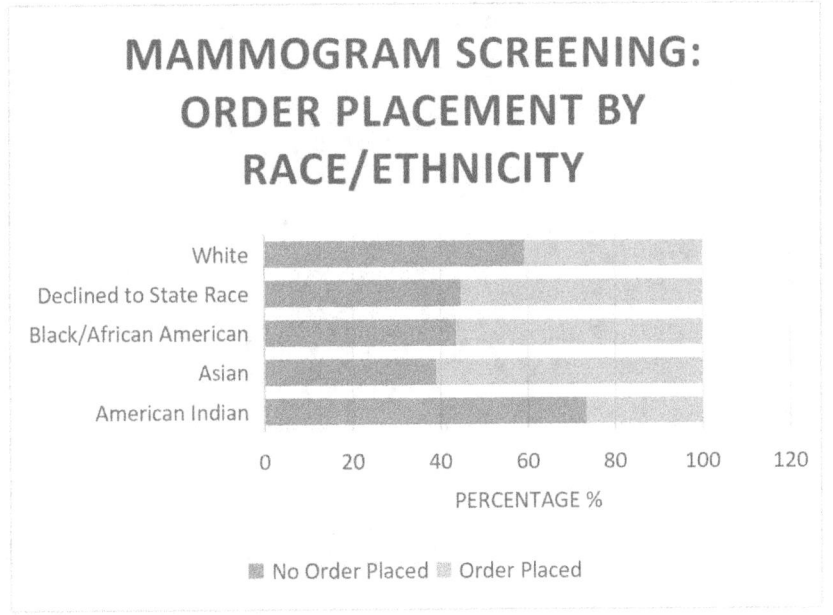

2. Prostate Cancer Screening Gaps

A similar analysis of **prostate-specific antigen (PSA) order rates** for male patients aged 55-69 uncovered disparities in screening for prostate cancer. Among the **23,984 eligible patients** who had seen a primary care physician (PCP), **37%** did not have a PSA order, and racial disparities were evident in the PSA order rates.

This is particularly concerning for high-risk groups such as **African American men** and those with a family history of prostate cancer or genetic predispositions like BRCA1/2 mutations. While completion rates for PSA screening were high at 91% across different racial and ethnic groups once the test was ordered, the significant gap in PSA orders indicates that some patients may not be receiving adequate preventive care.

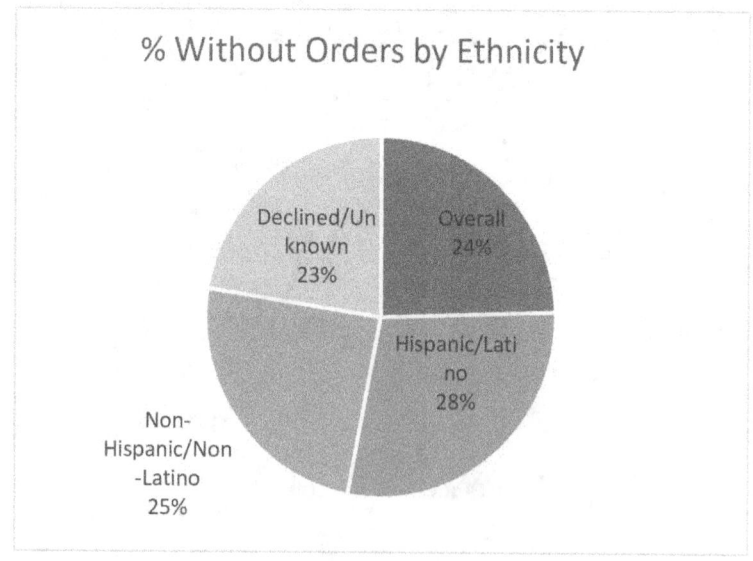

Stanford has introduced solutions such as **SmartPhrase**, a tool integrated into the **electronic health record (EHR)**, which helps track prostate screening and shared decision-making discussions between patients and providers. This enables clinicians to better document PSA screenings and ensures that at-risk populations are more likely to be offered and complete screening. Additionally, **education sessions** for providers have been rolled out to improve knowledge and practices related to prostate cancer screening, helping to close the gap in order rates and ensuring equitable access to care.

3. Tackling Lung Cancer Screening Disparities

Lung cancer screening (LCS) data reveal additional disparities in access to life-saving diagnostic services. From January 1, 2023, to July 25, 2024, data showed that racial and ethnic minorities, particularly **Black or African American patients**, were underrepresented in lung cancer screening completion rates. Given the disproportionate burden of lung cancer in marginalized communities, this gap raises critical questions about access to and utilization of LCS services.

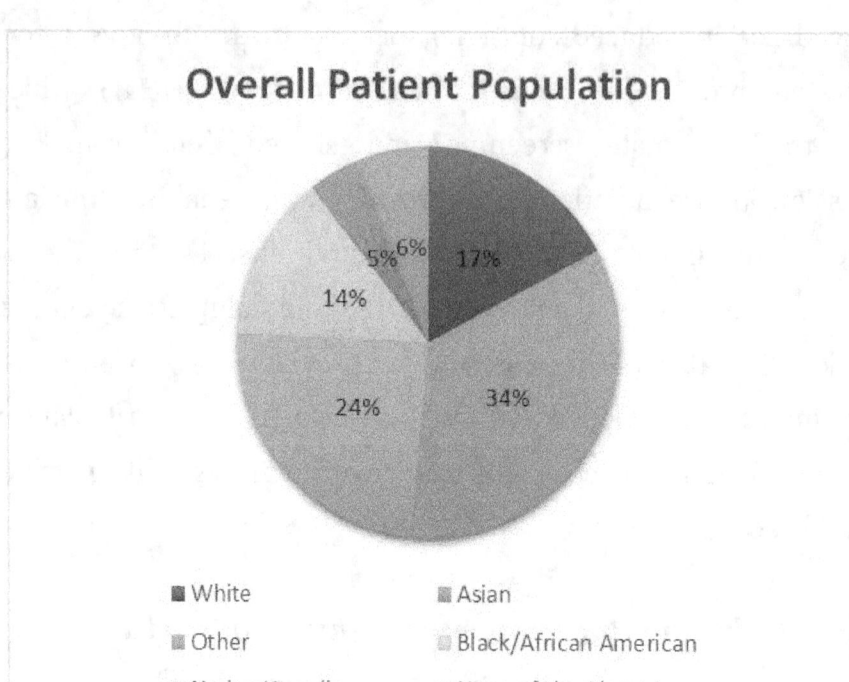

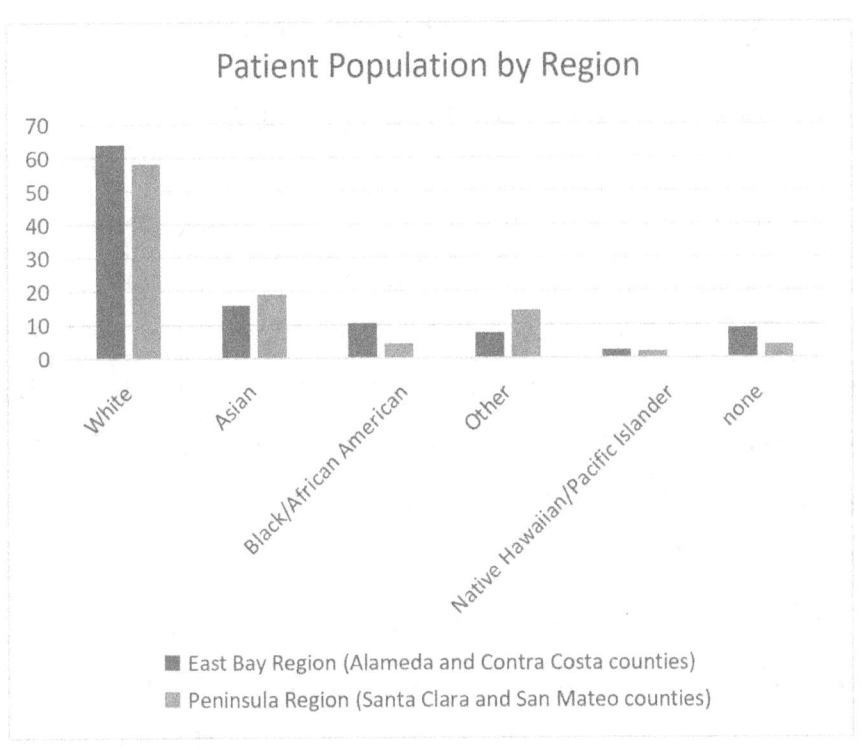

Stanford is focused on implementing **community outreach programs** and targeted interventions aimed at increasing awareness and participation in lung cancer screening, particularly among underrepresented groups. The objective is to improve trust between healthcare providers and patients from diverse backgrounds, foster culturally competent care, and enhance access to preventive screening programs. Efforts include expanding mobile imaging services and providing transportation support to remove logistical barriers that prevent patients from completing lung cancer screenings.

4. Health Equity Initiatives and Future Strategies

Stanford Medicine's efforts to promote health equity in radiology extend beyond individual screenings. The hospital is actively working to incorporate **cultural competency training** for radiologists and technologists to ensure that all staff members are equipped to interact with patients from diverse cultural backgrounds in a respectful and effective manner. This training covers everything from understanding cultural health beliefs to addressing language barriers, all of which can affect patient engagement and outcomes.

In addition to education, Stanford is also investing in **community-based research** that explores the impact of social determinants of health (SDOH) on access to imaging services. By studying how factors like income, education, and neighborhood environments influence health outcomes, Stanford is better positioned to tailor its interventions to the specific needs of the communities it serves.

One of the hospital's primary goals is to increase the **representation of underrepresented minorities in clinical trials** and research related to radiology. This includes outreach to Black, Hispanic, and other minority populations who have historically been excluded from medical research, ensuring that future diagnostic tools and treatments are effective across all demographic groups.

Stanford's leadership in **health equity research** and **patient advocacy** provides a framework for other healthcare institutions to follow. With continued focus on improving screening rates, expanding access to underserved populations, and addressing the unique challenges faced by diverse communities, Stanford is paving the way for a more equitable future in radiology and imaging.

Health equity in radiology at **Stanford Medicine** is an ongoing commitment to ensuring that every patient has access to high-quality, patient-centered imaging services, regardless of their background. By addressing disparities in breast, prostate, and lung cancer screenings, implementing community outreach, and advancing cultural competency within radiology practices, Stanford is setting the standard for equitable healthcare delivery. These efforts are crucial in reducing healthcare disparities, promoting inclusive care, and ultimately improving health outcomes for all patients.

Stanford Medicine's Frameworks and Models for Promoting Health Equity

Stanford Medicine is deeply committed to advancing health equity through a variety of frameworks, models, and programs that aim to provide equal access to high-quality healthcare services, including diagnostic imaging. These initiatives are designed to reduce health disparities, foster community partnerships, and promote a culture of diversity, equity, and inclusion (DEI) across all clinical practices. By leveraging innovative programs, technology, and research, Stanford is at the forefront of addressing the social determinants of health (SDOH) that contribute to disparities in healthcare.

1. *The Radiology Wellness Screening Program*

The **Radiology Wellness Screening Program** is one of Stanford's cornerstone efforts to promote early detection and proactive health monitoring through comprehensive preventive screenings. These screenings target a wide range of health conditions, enabling patients to detect potential issues early and receive timely interventions, ultimately improving outcomes.

Key screenings in this program include:

- **CT Heart Calcium Score**:
    - **Purpose**: Measures calcium buildup in the heart's arteries to assess cardiovascular risk.
    - **Access**: Allows patients to take proactive steps toward managing their heart health by identifying risks early.
- **CT Lung Cancer Screening**:
    - **Purpose**: Detects early-stage lung cancer in at-risk populations.

- **Eligibility**: Based on **USPSTF 2021 Guidelines**, includes individuals aged 50-80 with a smoking history of at least 20 pack years.
- **Impact**: Ensures early detection, particularly critical for high-risk populations such as long-term smokers.

- **CT Virtual Colonoscopy Screening**:
  - **Purpose**: A non-invasive screening for colon cancer.
  - **Importance**: Provides an alternative to traditional colonoscopy, making it more accessible and less invasive.

- **Screening Automated Whole-Breast Ultrasound (SAWBU)**:
  - **Purpose**: Detects breast cancer, especially useful for women with dense breast tissue.
  - **Significance**: Offers a critical screening option for women who may not be effectively served by traditional mammograms.

These services empower patients to take ownership of their health through **preventive care**, reducing the likelihood of advanced-stage diagnoses and costly treatments. By offering self-pay options and insurance coverage for many services, the program ensures that financial barriers do not prevent individuals from accessing necessary screenings.

2. Stanford Health Care Cost Estimator

The **Stanford Health Care Cost Estimator** is an essential tool designed to help patients make informed financial decisions about their healthcare. This user-friendly online platform allows individuals to estimate out-of-pocket expenses for common procedures, imaging exams, and services, giving patients greater control over their healthcare finances.

Purpose: Helps patients navigate the cost of services and anticipate financial obligations, enabling them to make informed decisions about their care.

Impact: By providing transparency in healthcare costs, the tool promotes **financial accessibility** and reduces the risk of surprise medical bills, which are a common barrier to care for underinsured patients.

3. C-I-CARE Training

C-**I-CARE** (Cultivating Interactions and Compassion for Equity) is Stanford's signature training program designed to improve communication and compassion in patient interactions. This initiative emphasizes cultural competence, empathy, and equity to ensure all patients receive **respectful, patient-centered care**.

Key Elements:

- Enhances the ability of healthcare providers to interact effectively with patients from diverse backgrounds.

- Promotes the principles of **diversity, equity, and inclusion** (DEI) by embedding these values into everyday patient care.

- **Outcomes**: C-I-CARE fosters an inclusive environment where every patient feels valued, contributing to higher **patient satisfaction** and better overall health outcomes.

- **Annual training** and onboarding sessions for radiology staff ensure that compassionate care remains a central focus of the patient experience at Stanford.

4. *MyHealth App*

The **MyHealth App** provides patients with a **convenient, mobile-friendly platform** to manage all aspects of their healthcare. By facilitating seamless access to services, communication, and health information, this app reduces barriers to care, particularly for underserved populations.

Key Features:

- **Appointment Management**: Patients can schedule, reschedule, or cancel appointments directly from the app, improving accessibility and reducing no-show rates.

- **Lab and Imaging Results**: Provide real-time access to lab results and radiology images, empowering patients to stay informed about their health.

- **Secure Messaging**: Enhances communication between patients and care teams, ensuring timely responses to questions or follow-up care.

- **Medication Management**: Helps patients track prescriptions, request refills, and set reminders for medications, promoting adherence to treatment plans.

- **Telehealth Services**: Enables patients to access virtual care, reducing the need for in-person visits and improving healthcare access, particularly for patients with mobility or transportation challenges.

By giving patients greater control over their healthcare, the **MyHealth App** plays a pivotal role in promoting **equity** by making healthcare more accessible and patient-friendly, particularly for those facing traditional barriers to care.

5. *SPHERE and the HEAL Network*

The **Stanford Precision Health for Ethnic and Racial Equity (SPHERE)** Center, funded by the **National Institutes of Health (NIH)**, is a pioneering initiative that addresses health disparities through precision medicine. SPHERE's mission is to use precision health tools to improve the outcomes of **racially and**

ethnically diverse populations, traditionally underrepresented in clinical research.

HEAL Network: The **Network for Health Equity Action Leadership (HEAL)** is an extension of SPHERE that promotes **community engagement**, **research collaborations**, and **policy development** to reduce health disparities. It brings together experts and community members to create impactful change in minority health outcomes.

Outcomes:

- Engages communities in precision health research, addressing unique health challenges faced by minority populations.
- Advances healthcare equity by developing tailored interventions based on genomic, environmental, and social factors.

6. REACH Initiative

The **Racial Equity to Advance a Community of Health (REACH) Initiative** is another cornerstone of Stanford Medicine's equity efforts. This initiative seeks to cultivate a new generation of medical and scientific leaders who are committed to **social justice**, **racial equity**, and **health equity**.

Key Focus: Training and developing leaders who will champion equity within healthcare and beyond. Addressing the

severe health disparities that disproportionately affect minority populations, both locally and nationally.

7. Community Health and Partnerships Program

Stanford Health Care's **Community Health and Partnerships Program** is a comprehensive effort to improve community health outcomes, particularly for the most vulnerable populations. The program is informed by public health data and community feedback, ensuring that it targets the real needs of the communities it serves.

Key Initiatives:

- Conducts **community health needs assessments** every three years in collaboration with local health departments and residents.

- Provides over **$734.3 million** in community benefits in 2023, including funding for programs that address the healthcare needs of underserved populations.

- Works to improve **health equity** by addressing social determinants of health such as housing, food security, and access to care.

8. Radiology Diversity Initiative

The **Stanford Radiology Diversity Initiative** is dedicated to ensuring that the faculty and staff reflect the diversity of the communities they serve. By recruiting and retaining a **diverse workforce**, the initiative fosters an inclusive environment that promotes innovation, solves healthcare problems, and enhances patient care.

Goals:

- Create a **multicultural environment** where diverse perspectives and experiences drive better healthcare solutions.

- Support the development of culturally competent practices that address the unique needs of **multicultural patients**.

Stanford Medicine's frameworks and models for promoting health equity are at the forefront of creating an inclusive and equitable healthcare environment. From the **Radiology Wellness Screening Program** to the **REACH Initiative** and the **HEAL Network**, these programs represent Stanford's unwavering commitment to advancing healthcare access and equity for all. By leveraging cutting-edge technology, culturally competent care, and community engagement, Stanford Medicine continues to break down barriers to care and ensure that every patient has the opportunity to achieve optimal health.

Four (4) Key Takeaways

1. **Radiology's Role in Perpetuating Health Disparities:** Radiology has historically played a role in perpetuating healthcare disparities due to systemic inequities in access to imaging services. The underrepresentation of minority radiologists and unequal access to diagnostic technologies have contributed to poorer health outcomes for marginalized communities, particularly African Americans. These disparities reflect broader social inequities that have existed in healthcare for decades.

2. **Historical Inequities in Access to Imaging for African Americans:** African Americans have faced significant barriers to accessing radiology services throughout history, rooted in institutional racism and discriminatory practices. For example, in the 1960s, Black patients were subjected to higher radiation doses based on pseudoscientific beliefs, exposing them to greater health risks. These practices highlight the ongoing need to eliminate biases in medical procedures and ensure equitable care for all patients.

3. **The Path to Equity Through Lessons from History:** Learning from the harmful effects of using race as a proxy for biological differences in radiology, the field has taken steps to rectify these past injustices. Innovations like the ALARA principle and Automatic Exposure Control (AEC) have

improved patient safety and created more equitable imaging standards. By acknowledging historical mistakes, radiology can develop practices that treat patients as individuals, not racial categories.

4. **Innovation and Progress in Reducing Radiation Exposure:** Stanford Health Care has been a leader in pioneering new methods to minimize radiation exposure for all patients. Advances in imaging technology, such as cumulative dose tracking, have significantly improved patient safety and reduced disparities in care. These innovations, alongside efforts to monitor and reduce radiation exposure in at-risk populations, demonstrate Stanford's commitment to equitable healthcare delivery.

SECTION 3

CASE STUDIES ADDRESSING SOCIAL AND COMMUNITY CONTEXT IN RADIOLOGY

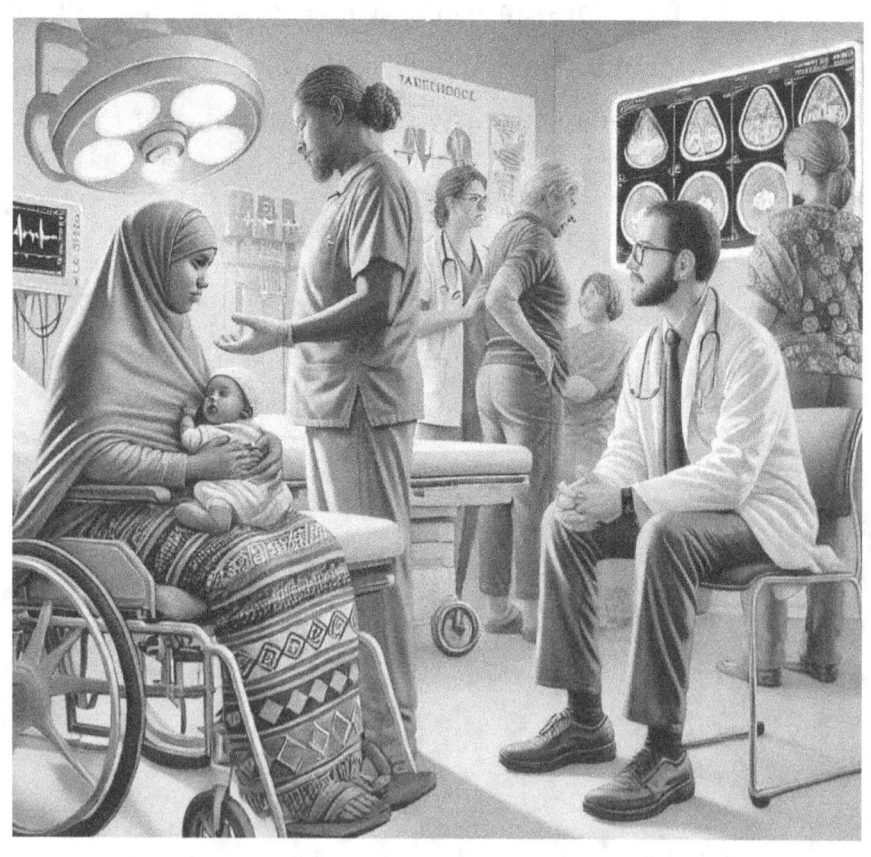

1. Case Study 1: Social and Community Context

A Comprehensive Strategy for SDOH

Addressing social determinants of health (SDOH) in radiology requires a flexible, patient-centered approach that integrates program support, resource allocation, and collaboration between healthcare providers and communities. This case study highlights how healthcare providers, particularly in radiology, can apply cultural sensitivity and personalized care to improve patient outcomes. By considering the unique social and community context of each patient, healthcare teams can deliver more effective and compassionate care.

Patient Profile

Ms. Amina, a 35-year-old Somali immigrant, presents with persistent abdominal pain and bloating. She works part-time as a housekeeper, supporting a family of six, including four children under the age of ten. Her limited English proficiency, cultural and religious beliefs about healthcare, and responsibilities as a caregiver have contributed to her delayed seeking of medical attention. Due to her symptoms, an ultrasound examination is ordered to evaluate a potential ovarian cyst.

Challenges:

- Cultural barriers: Ms. Amina's religious and cultural practices may impact her comfort with healthcare services, including a preference for same-gender providers.

- Language barriers: Limited English proficiency hinders her ability to fully understand her condition and the treatment options available.

- Social context: As the primary caregiver for four young children, Ms. Amina may face logistical challenges attending appointments and seeking care.

- Opportunity: By addressing her cultural, linguistic, and social needs, the radiology team has the opportunity to significantly improve her care experience, ensuring that she receives timely and respectful treatment.

Engaging Ms. Amina: Pertinent Questions for Personalized Care

These tailored questions will help the radiology team better understand Ms. Amina's unique circumstances and cultural context, allowing for more personalized and effective care:

- **Would you prefer same-gender healthcare providers for your comfort?**

Understanding her cultural preferences regarding gender may help alleviate anxiety during the examination.

- **Can you share more about your support network?**

   This question helps the care team assess the role of her family and community in providing emotional and logistical support.

- **Are there any cultural or religious practices related to your health that we should be aware of?**

   Cultural sensitivity is crucial to ensure the patient feels respected and that her beliefs are incorporated into her care.

- **Do you feel comfortable communicating in English, or would you prefer an interpreter?**

   Offering an interpreter allows Ms. Amina to better understand her diagnosis and treatment options, empowering her to make informed decisions.

- **Do you have any concerns about the use of ultrasound technology in diagnosis?**

   Addressing potential fears about medical technology from a cultural perspective may help reduce anxiety and improve cooperation during the exam.

- **Would you like to discuss the ultrasound findings with your family, or would you prefer to keep the information confidential?**

  Respecting the patient's privacy preferences builds trust and strengthens the patient-provider relationship.

- **Are there any other language or cultural nuances we should be aware of to ensure your comfort?**

  This open-ended question allows Ms. Amina to express any additional needs that may not have been addressed.

Next Steps for the Radiology Team: Culturally Sensitive Care

To ensure that Ms. Amina receives the best possible care, the radiology team should take the following steps:

- Cultural Sensitivity Intervention:
  Involve a female Somali interpreter during her consultation to facilitate understanding and respect her cultural preferences. This will help Ms. Amina feel comfortable, ensuring she can fully grasp her condition and treatment options.

- Patient Education with Visual Aids:
  Deliver educational materials that incorporate **visual aids** and are communicated at an educational level suited to Ms.

Amina's comprehension. This approach helps bridge language gaps and ensures that important medical information is understood.

- Logistical Support:
Offer assistance in arranging childcare or providing flexible appointment times, acknowledging her role as a caregiver. This will enable Ms. Amina to focus on her health without added stress from her family responsibilities.

Communication and Support for Ms. Amina

The following communication approaches and statements can be utilized by the radiology team to foster trust and engagement with Ms. Amina:

- Cultural Sensitivity and Communication:

"We respect and value your unique cultural and religious beliefs. Please share any preferences or concerns you have so that we can provide the best care possible. Your comfort and understanding are our top priorities."

- Language Support and Interpretation Services:

"We provide interpretation services to ensure clear communication during your ultrasound. Let us know if you would like assistance in your native language, and we'll

make the necessary arrangements to accommodate your needs."

- Family Support and Care Coordination:

"We understand that managing your family's needs is important. Let us know if we can help you arrange for childcare during your visit or if there are other ways we can assist."

- Patient Empowerment and Education:

"Your health and well-being are important to us. We will take the time to explain everything clearly and answer any questions you may have. Please don't hesitate to ask if anything is unclear."

- Personalized Care and Support:

"We know that seeking medical help can sometimes be difficult, but we are here to support you every step of the way. Your health is our priority, and we are dedicated to making sure you feel cared for and understood."

Conclusion: Enhancing Radiology Practices through Cultural Sensitivity

This case study illustrates the critical importance of incorporating **social and community context** into radiology practices. By understanding and addressing Ms. Amina's cultural, linguistic, and social needs, the radiology team can significantly improve her care experience. **Cultural sensitivity**, **communication support**, and **personalized care** are essential in ensuring that patients from diverse backgrounds receive the attention, respect, and care they deserve.

Stanford Healthcare Radiology and radiology teams across healthcare systems can improve healthcare outcomes by integrating cultural competency, addressing social determinants of health, and fostering trust within communities. Ensuring that radiology practices consider **patients' cultural contexts** is a vital step toward achieving health equity and improving patient satisfaction.

Educational Resources for Immigrants, Refugees, Asylees, and Other New Americans

For further support, the U.S. Department of Education offers valuable information and resources tailored to immigrant and refugee families. Visit: U.S. Department of Education Resources for Immigrants and Refugees

2. Case Study 2: Economic Stability in Radiology

A Comprehensive Approach to Economic Barriers in Healthcare

Effectively addressing social determinants of health (SDOH) requires a flexible strategy that combines program support, resource allocation, and collaboration between healthcare providers and communities. This case study illustrates how radiology staff can recognize and mitigate economic barriers, ensuring equitable access to essential diagnostic services for patients facing financial challenges.

Patient Profile

Maria Gonzalez is a 48-year-old single mother of two children, ages 10 and 12. She works part-time as a cashier at a local grocery store, relying on public transportation for her daily commute. Maria's monthly income barely covers basic necessities such as rent, utilities, and food. She depends on Medicaid for her healthcare needs but often struggles with co-pays and out-of-pocket expenses.

Maria has a history of hypertension and type 2 diabetes, both of which require regular monitoring and medication. Recently, she has been experiencing persistent headaches and visual disturbances. During a visit to her primary care physician (PCP), her blood pressure and blood glucose levels were found to be significantly elevated. Concerned about potential complications, her PCP refers her for a brain MRI to rule out any neurological issues.

Challenges

- Financial Constraints: Limited income makes it difficult for Maria to afford medications, co-pays, and other healthcare-related expenses.

- Transportation Barriers: Reliance on public transportation may cause delays or difficulties in reaching medical appointments.

- Work Schedule Conflicts: As a part-time employee without paid leave, missing work for appointments could result in lost wages or job insecurity.

- Childcare Responsibilities: Managing childcare during medical appointments adds another layer of complexity.

Opportunity

By understanding Maria's economic and social challenges, the radiology team can implement strategies to alleviate these barriers, ensuring she receives the necessary diagnostic care without additional stress.

Engaging Maria: Pertinent Questions for Personalized Support

To better understand Maria's situation and provide appropriate assistance, the radiology staff can ask:

- **"Do you have any concerns about taking time off work for your medical appointments?"**

  This identifies potential scheduling conflicts and financial implications.

- **"Is your current income sufficient to meet your basic needs, including healthcare costs?"**

  This helps assess financial strain and eligibility for assistance programs.

- **"Are you experiencing any difficulties affording medications or other healthcare-related expenses?"**

  This opens the door to discuss medication assistance or alternative options.

- **"Do you have reliable transportation to get to and from your medical appointments?"**

  This identifies transportation barriers that may prevent her from attending appointments.

- **"Would you like information on transportation assistance programs that can help you get to your appointments?"**

  This offers practical solutions to overcome transportation issues.

- **"Do you have family or friends who can help with childcare when you have medical appointments?"**

  This assesses her support network for managing childcare responsibilities.

- **"Are there any community resources or support networks you rely on for assistance?"**

  This identifies existing support systems that can be leveraged.

- **"Do you have any concerns about accessing follow-up care or additional treatments recommended by your healthcare providers?"**

  Uncovers potential barriers to ongoing care.

- **"Have you experienced any barriers to receiving the medical care you need?"**

  This provides an opportunity for Maria to share any other challenges she faces.

- **"Do you feel comfortable understanding the medical information and instructions provided by your healthcare team?"**

    This assesses health literacy and the need for additional communication support.

- **"Do you understand the purpose of the MRI and the potential next steps depending on the results?"**

    This ensures she is informed about the procedure and its importance.

Next Steps for the Radiology Team: Providing Comprehensive Support

- Scheduling Flexibility
    - Offer Evening or Weekend Appointments: To minimize disruption to her work schedule and reduce the risk of lost wages.
    - Streamline Appointments: Coordinate with other departments to consolidate appointments when possible.

- Transportation Assistance

    o Provide Information on Transportation Services: Share details about free patient shuttles or programs offering transportation assistance for medical appointments.

    o Assist in Arranging Transportation: Help schedule rides if necessary.

- Financial Counseling

    o Connect with a Social Worker or Financial Counselor: Arrange a meeting to discuss her financial concerns and explore options such as sliding scale fees or payment plans.

    o Guide Through Assistance Programs: Help her apply for additional support programs like medication assistance or local aid.

- Medication Assistance

    o Explore Generic Alternatives: Coordinate with her healthcare provider to consider more affordable medication options.

    o Investigate Manufacturer Assistance Programs: Check for available coupons or programs that reduce medication costs.

- Childcare Support

    o   Provide Resources: Offer information on community organizations that provide childcare assistance during medical appointments.

- Clear Communication

    o   Simplify Medical Information: Use plain language and visual aids to explain the MRI procedure and ensure she understands the importance of follow-up care.

    o   Verify Understanding: Encourage her to ask questions and repeat information back to confirm comprehension.

Communication Strategies: Supporting Maria with Empathy

a. Financial Assistance and Resources

"At Stanford Radiology, we can guide you in exploring our specialized financial assistance programs designed to help patients manage healthcare costs effectively."

"Some medication manufacturers offer assistance programs that could lower your out-of-pocket costs. We can check if such programs are available for your prescriptions."

"Let's review your health insurance coverage together to ensure you're getting the maximum benefits and explore options to optimize your coverage for healthcare services."

b. Transportation Support

"We understand that transportation can be challenging. We offer free patient shuttles between various Stanford Health Care locations. Would you like information on how to use these services?"

"If public transportation isn't convenient, there are local programs that provide transportation assistance for medical appointments. We can help you connect with them."

c. Scheduling Assistance

"We want to make your appointment as convenient as possible. Are there specific days or times that work best for you? We have evening and weekend slots available."

d. Childcare Resources

"Managing childcare can be difficult during medical visits. We can provide information on community resources that offer childcare support if that would be helpful."

e. Empowering Patient Engagement

"Your health is important to us, and we're here to support you. Please let us know if you have any concerns or questions about your MRI or any other aspect of your care."

"We want to ensure that you fully understand the procedure and what to expect. Feel free to ask any questions, and we'll provide all the information you need."

Conclusion: Bridging Economic Barriers in Radiology

With the support of hospital resources and compassionate care from the radiology team, Maria can navigate her medical and economic challenges more effectively. This case study highlights the critical intersection of economic stability and access to radiological services. By offering flexible scheduling, transportation assistance, and financial counseling, healthcare providers can significantly mitigate the economic barriers faced by low-income patients like Maria. This comprehensive support not only improves health outcomes but also contributes to the overall well-being of patients struggling with economic instability.

Resources for Patients Facing Economic Challenges

- Stanford Health Care Financial Counseling
    - Services: Offers financial assistance options for uninsured and underinsured patients. Counseling helps patients explore programs to cover medical costs or qualify for financial aid.
    - Contacts:

- Palo Alto: 650.498.2900
- Tri-Valley: 925.534.6457
- More Information: <u>Stanford Health Care Financial Counseling</u>

- Stanford Medicine Transportation Services
    - Services: Provides transportation assistance for patients needing help getting to and from medical appointments, including free patient shuttles between Stanford Health Care locations. Specialized transportation for patients requiring wheelchair-accessible vehicles is also coordinated.
    - Contact: TransportationServices@stanfordhealthcare.org or 650.736.8000
    - Information: Free transportation is available for patients and visitors between key Stanford Health Care facilities.

- Stanford Health Care Navigation Bar
    - Services: Enhances the patient experience by offering support with MyHealth enrollment, referrals for billing questions, financial aid, and information on housing and accommodations.
    - Contact: 650.497.6426
    - Explore: <u>Stanford Health Care Navigation Bar</u>

- Temporary Assistance for Needy Families (TANF)
    - Services: Provides financial assistance and support services to low-income families with children to promote economic self-sufficiency.
    - Access: <u>Temporary Assistance for Needy Families</u>
- CareerOneStop
    - Services: Offers career-related tools and resources for job seekers, students, and employers, including job search assistance and training programs.
    - Website: <u>CareerOneStop</u>
- U.S. Housing and Urban Development (HUD)
    - Services: Identifies local nonprofit organizations offering housing assistance, provides guidance on foreclosure prevention, and helps find regional housing authorities.
    - Explore: <u>U.S. HUD</u>
- ApprenticeshipUSA
    - Services: Supports the development of accessible Registered Apprenticeship opportunities, benefiting workers seeking advanced positions.
    - Details: <u>ApprenticeshipUSA</u>

- ClearPoint Credit Counseling Solutions

    Services: A non-profit organization offering financial counseling and education services to individuals in need.
    Visit: [ClearPoint Credit Counseling Solutions](#)

By providing these resources and personalized support, the radiology team can help patients like Maria overcome economic challenges, ensuring they receive the necessary medical care without undue hardship. This approach fosters health equity, enabling all patients to access essential healthcare services regardless of their financial situation.

3. Case Study 3: Addressing Education Access and Quality in Radiology

A Holistic Approach to Overcoming Health Literacy Barriers in Diagnostic Care

Effectively addressing social determinants of health (SDOH) requires healthcare providers to consider the impact of education access and quality on a patient's ability to navigate medical care. This case study illustrates how radiology staff can support a patient with limited health literacy, ensuring clear communication, culturally appropriate care, and thorough education about their condition and treatment options.

Patient Profile

Mr. Wozniak, a 50-year-old manual laborer originally from Poland, presents at Stanford Health Care with persistent and intense pain in his right foot after accidentally dropping a heavy object at work. Despite the pain, Mr. Wozniak delayed seeking medical attention due to his belief that the injury would resolve on its own. With a limited educational background (having only completed middle school) and low health literacy, Mr. Wozniak struggled to recognize the severity of his condition.

His primary care physician (PCP) has now referred him for an X-ray to confirm suspected fractures, and the radiology team plays a crucial role in ensuring that Mr. Wozniak understands the importance of timely diagnosis and treatment.

Challenges

Limited Health Literacy: Mr. Wozniak's low health literacy has led to delayed care and a lack of understanding about the seriousness of his injury.

Language Barriers: Mr. Wozniak is a Polish speaker with limited proficiency in English, making it difficult for him to navigate the healthcare system and understand medical instructions.

Physical Demands of Work: As a manual laborer, his job is physically demanding, and his ability to work may be compromised due to the injury.

Opportunity

By addressing Mr. Wozniak's health literacy and language needs, the radiology team can ensure he receives the care he requires in a timely manner while also empowering him to take control of his healthcare decisions.

Engaging Mr. Wozniak: Pertinent Questions for Personalized Support

To gain a better understanding of Mr. Wozniak's situation and provide comprehensive support, the radiology staff can ask:

- **"How severe would you rate your pain on a scale of 1 to 10, with 10 being the most severe?"**

    This helps the staff assess the urgency of the injury and Mr. Wozniak's pain level.

- **"Have you ever had an X-ray? Is there anything you would like to know about this process?"**

    This offers an opportunity to explain the procedure in simple terms and address any fears or concerns he may have.

- **"Can you tell us about any worries or reservations you have about the treatment process?"**

    This ensures that his emotional and cultural concerns are addressed before proceeding with the exam.

- **"Can you manage to visit us for follow-up X-rays and consultations, given your work schedule?"**

    This helps the team plan around his work commitments to avoid further delays in care.

- **"Can you describe the nature of your job? Is it physically demanding? Will your injury interfere with your ability to work?"**

    This offers insight into how his injury might impact his livelihood and informs further treatment plans.

- **"Do you feel well-informed about managing your health?"**

    This opens a dialogue to assess his understanding of general health management and the importance of prompt medical care.

Next Steps for the Radiology Team: Comprehensive Support

- **Patient Education**
    - Simplify Medical Information: The radiology team should use simple language and visual aids to explain the X-ray findings and the importance of following through with treatment.

- Clarify Treatment Steps: Ensure that Mr. Wozniak fully understands the potential need for immobilization and follow-up care, emphasizing how these steps will support his recovery.

- **Coordination with Other Healthcare Providers**
    - Collaborate with Orthopedic and PCP Teams: The radiology staff should keep in close contact with Mr. Wozniak's orthopedic specialist and PCP to ensure continuity of care. If unusual findings arise during follow-up X-rays, they should be promptly communicated to the wider care team.
    - Assist with Scheduling: Help coordinate follow-up appointments that fit within Mr. Wozniak's work schedule to avoid disruption to his livelihood.

- **Evaluate Systemic Issues**
    - Investigate Occupational Risks: If Mr. Wozniak's injury hints at a broader systemic issue (e.g., unsafe working conditions), the healthcare team should consider collaborating with occupational health services or public health authorities to address potential workplace hazards.

Supporting Mr. Wozniak: Key Statements for Clear Communication

Patient Education and Explanation

"We understand that seeking medical care can sometimes be overwhelming, especially with unfamiliar procedures like X-rays. We're here to help. We'll walk you through every step, explaining how the X-ray will help diagnose your injury and what the results mean."

"If you have any questions or concerns about your foot injury or the X-ray process, feel free to ask. We want to make sure you're comfortable and well-informed."

Instructions and Guidance in Polish

"To ensure you fully understand the procedure and treatment, we can provide educational materials and explanations in Polish. Please let us know if that would help you feel more comfortable."

"We will guide you through the X-ray process step by step and provide clear instructions in Polish so you can feel confident during your visit."

Language Support for Communication

"We can arrange for a Polish interpreter during your visit to help make sure you understand all aspects of your care. It's important that you feel heard and comfortable."

Interpretation of Diagnostic Results

"After we review the results of your X-ray, we'll explain any findings—such as fractures—so you know exactly what's going on with your injury. We'll make sure to explain everything in Polish, if that's easier for you."

Assistance with Healthcare Literacy

"Our team is here to help you navigate any medical information you need to understand. We want to ensure you feel empowered to make informed decisions about your care."

Conclusion: Bridging Education Gaps in Radiology

Given Mr. Wozniak's limited education and health literacy, it is essential that the radiology team pays extra attention to simplifying explanations, providing clear instructions, and addressing his language needs. This case study highlights the importance of considering education access and quality when delivering healthcare, especially in radiology. Ensuring Mr. Wozniak understands his diagnosis and treatment plan is crucial for his recovery and for preventing future delays in care. With compassionate, culturally sensitive communication, the healthcare team can empower Mr. Wozniak to take an active role in his health, leading to better outcomes.

Resources for Supporting Patients with Limited Education and Language Barriers

- Stanford Health Care Interpreter Services
    - Services: Offers free medical interpretation and translation services for patients needing language support during in-person, video, or telephone appointments.
    - Contact: 650.723.6940 OR 650.497.7780
    - More Information: <u>Interpreter Services at Stanford Health Care</u>

- Stanford Health Care International Medical Services
    - Services: Provides comprehensive medical and financial orientations for international patients to help them navigate the healthcare system and understand their treatment options.
    - Contact: 650.723.8561
    - More Information: <u>International Medical Services at Stanford Health Care</u>

- Stanford Hospital Health Library
    - Services: Access a wide range of scientifically based health information to guide informed decisions and receive culturally competent health education services free.

- Contact: 650.725.8400
- More Information: Stanford Hospital Health Library

- MyHealthFinder
    - Services: An evidence-based wellness tool recommended by health professionals, offering health information in English and Spanish for individuals and families.
    - Explore: MyHealthFinder

- U.S. Department of Education
    - Services: Provides resources designed for students, parents, and educators to facilitate education outside traditional classroom settings, supporting lifelong learning.
    - Explore: U.S. Department of Education Resources

By addressing Mr. Wozniak's unique needs through clear communication, language support, and tailored educational resources, the radiology team ensures that he receives the care he needs while empowering him to be actively engaged in his treatment plan. This patient-centered approach promotes health equity by acknowledging and addressing the social factors that impact health outcomes, ensuring that all patients, regardless of their education level or language, have access to quality healthcare.

4. Case Study 4: Addressing Food Insecurity and Health in Diagnostic Imaging

A Comprehensive Approach to Navigating Nutritional Barriers and Healthcare Access

In this case study, the radiology team works with a patient facing significant food insecurity, highlighting the critical need for holistic care that addresses both medical and social determinants of health (SDOH). By understanding John Smith's economic challenges and how they influence his overall well-being, the radiology team can offer tailored support that leads to better health outcomes.

Patient Profile

John Smith, a 52-year-old man with a history of hypertension, chronic fatigue, and unexplained weight loss, has been experiencing severe fatigue and occasional palpitations over the past six months. Despite managing his conditions with over-the-counter medications and lifestyle changes, his symptoms have persisted. John relies on Medicaid for healthcare and utilizes food banks and Supplemental Nutrition Assistance Program (SNAP) benefits to manage food insecurity.

Due to his worsening symptoms, his primary care physician (PCP) suspects thyroid dysfunction and refers him for a nuclear medicine thyroid scan to evaluate thyroid function.

Challenges

Food Insecurity: John's reliance on food banks and SNAP benefits indicates that he may struggle to maintain a consistent, nutritious diet, which could exacerbate his health conditions.

Limited Financial Resources: His dependence on Medicaid and other support programs suggests financial strain that might hinder access to care and medications.

Health Literacy and Engagement: John's limited access to proper nutrition and healthcare might have contributed to delays in seeking medical help, impacting his ability to manage his chronic conditions effectively.

Opportunity

By addressing John's food insecurity alongside his medical needs, the radiology and nuclear medicine team can provide a more comprehensive care plan that improves both his thyroid health and his overall nutritional status. The team can empower John with knowledge, resources, and support systems that address the root causes of his persistent health issues.

Engaging John Smith: Pertinent Questions for Personalized Support.

To gain a deeper understanding of John's situation and identify potential barriers, the radiology staff can ask the following questions:

- **"Do you have enough food to maintain a balanced diet, or do you often find yourself without enough to eat?"**

  This question opens the door to understanding how food insecurity might be affecting his overall health and well-being.

- **"Are there days when you skip meals because you can't afford to buy food?**

  Uncovering the extent of his food insecurity can help the team assess the urgency of connecting him to food assistance resources.

- **"Are you facing any financial difficulties that make it hard to pay for your medications or other healthcare needs?"**

  John's financial struggles will allow the team to explore potential assistance programs for medication and healthcare services.

- **"How do you usually travel to your medical appointments?"**

  Identifying transportation barriers will help the team provide solutions, such as transportation assistance programs or flexible scheduling.

- **"Is there anything preventing you from accessing the medical care you need, such as cost or lack of support?"**

  This question enables the team to uncover other obstacles that might be impacting John's ability to prioritize his health.

- **"Would it be helpful for you to speak with a financial counselor or social worker to explore additional resources?"**

  Offering financial counseling and social support can help John navigate his financial and health-related challenges more effectively.

- **"Do you understand the results of your thyroid scan and the treatment options available to you?"**

  Ensuring that John comprehends his medical condition and treatment plan will empower him to take control of his healthcare decisions.

- "Would you like additional information on how to manage hyperthyroidism, including dietary advice?"

Providing nutritional guidance, especially given his food insecurity, can help John make the most of the resources available to him.

Next Steps for the Radiology Team: Comprehensive Support

- Scheduling Flexibility

Accommodate John's Work Schedule: To minimize disruptions and ensure he can attend appointments, the radiology team can schedule his nuclear medicine thyroid scan during off-hours or provide transportation options if needed.

- Nutritional Support

Referral to a Dietitian: The radiology team should connect John with a hospital dietitian to create a nutritional plan that fits within his financial limitations. This plan can help him optimize his diet to support his thyroid health, even with limited resources.

Connect with Local Food Assistance Programs: The team can also guide John to food assistance programs that provide access to nutritious meals, such as community food banks and meal services designed for individuals facing food insecurity.

- Financial Counseling

    Engage a Social Worker: A social worker can meet with John to discuss additional support programs, such as Medicaid benefits, prescription assistance, and other financial resources that could help him manage healthcare costs and improve his access to medications.

Supporting John Smith: Key Statements for Clear Communication

- Food Insecurity Resources

    "We understand that food insecurity can have a significant impact on your health. We can provide you with information about local food banks, community pantries, and programs that offer immediate food assistance to help support you during this time."

- Community Support for Nutrition

    "Our community health clinics work closely with social workers and nutritionists who can help you navigate food insecurity challenges. We'll connect you with these resources to ensure you have the support you need to maintain your nutrition and overall health."

- Transportation Assistance for Food Access

   "If transportation is a challenge, let us know. We can help explore transportation options or refer you to programs that offer services for food shopping or accessing other food support resources."

- Patient-Centered Nutrition Education

   "In addition to your medical care, we want to empower you to manage your food insecurity through education and resources. We can offer guidance on budget-friendly meal planning and making healthy choices within your financial limitations."

Conclusion: A Holistic Approach to Managing Health and Food Insecurity

With the appropriate support from the radiology team, John will be able to manage both his thyroid condition and his nutritional needs more effectively. By offering scheduling flexibility, nutritional counseling, and financial guidance, the team can address the significant barriers caused by his food insecurity, ensuring that John receives comprehensive care that improves his overall health and well-being.

Resources for Supporting Patients Facing Food Insecurity

- Stanford Health Care Outpatient Nutrition Services at Tri-Valley
    - Services: Offers customized nutrition plans, advanced treatment options, and comprehensive support for patients facing nutritional challenges.
    - Contact: 925.416.6720
    - More Information: <u>Outpatient Nutrition Services at Tri-Valley</u>
- Second Harvest Food Bank of Silicon Valley
    - Services: Distributes food through over 900 sites across Santa Clara and San Mateo counties. Programs include Lean Proteins for Local Food Distribution Centers and COVID-19 Relief Donations.
    - Contact: 1.800.984.3663
    - More Information: <u>Second Harvest Food Bank of Silicon Valley</u>
- Open Heart Food Bank
    - Services: Provides food distribution in the Tri-Valley area through programs such as Hot Meals, Senior Meal, and Street Outreach Programs.
    - Contact: 925.255.1225

- More Information: <u>Open Heart Food Bank</u>
- Supplemental Nutrition Assistance Program (SNAP)
  - Services: Provides food benefits to low-income families, helping them access nutritious food and manage grocery budgets.
  - More Information: <u>SNAP</u>
- Feeding America
  - Services: A national network of food banks dedicated to providing food access and addressing hunger concerns throughout the country.
  - More Information: <u>Feeding America</u>
- Women, Infants, and Children (WIC)
  - Services: A federal program supporting low-income women, infants, and children with nutrition assistance.
  - More Information: <u>Women, Infants, and Children (WIC)</u>
- USDA National Hunger Hotline
  - Services: Provides information about federal nutrition assistance programs through a toll-free telephone service in both English and Spanish.
  - Contact: 1-866-3-HUNGRY (1-866-348-6479) OR 1-877-8-HAMBRE (1-877-842-6273) for Spanish

By addressing both John's medical and social needs, the radiology team helps remove barriers to care, ensuring he receives the necessary support to manage his thyroid health and improve his nutritional well-being. This patient-centered approach not only enhances the quality of care but also contributes to health equity by addressing the complex social drivers impacting John's health.

5. *Case Study 5: Neighborhood and Built/Physical Environment*

Navigating Environmental Challenges and Healthcare Access in Rural Areas

A Comprehensive Approach to Addressing Health and Social Barriers for Mr. Juan

In this case study, the radiology team must consider the unique environmental and logistical challenges faced by Mr. Juan, who lives in a remote, rural area with limited access to healthcare services. His case study highlights the importance of understanding the intersection of environmental conditions, occupational exposure, and health equity. By addressing barriers such as transportation, access to nutritious food, and the financial constraints associated with low-income housing, the healthcare team can offer a more personalized and supportive care experience for Mr. Juan.

Patient Profile

Mr. Juan, a 60-year-old man from a rural area in Modesto, California, spent several years working in construction, which may have exposed him to asbestos and other hazardous materials. He lives in a low-income neighborhood with limited access to nutritious food, clean water, and recreational areas. Recently, he began experiencing severe coughing and shortness of breath, which prompted his primary care physician (PCP) to suspect lung disease related to his occupational exposure. Mr. Juan has been referred for a lung CT scan at Stanford's radiology department, but he faces transportation challenges and financial constraints that may impact his ability to receive care.

Understanding Mr. Juan's Situation: Pertinent Questions for Tailored Support

To provide personalized care and uncover potential barriers Mr. Juan may face, the radiology team can ask the following questions:

- **"Can you describe your living situation? Do you live in a housing complex, and what are the environmental conditions like?"**

    This question helps the team understand the physical and environmental factors that could be contributing to Mr.

Juan's health condition, such as mold, poor air quality, or exposure to toxins.

- **"Are there any activities or environmental factors that make your symptoms better or worse?"**

   By identifying triggers or mitigating factors, the team can tailor recommendations to Mr. Juan's lifestyle and environment.

- **"Have you previously undergone any diagnostic procedures or treatments for these symptoms?"**

   This helps assess his previous healthcare access and potential delays in diagnosis or treatment due to living in a remote area.

- **"Have you or anyone in your family been diagnosed with lung disease or other pulmonary conditions?"**

   This question provides insight into Mr. Juan's family health history and could reveal hereditary conditions or shared environmental exposures.

- **"Do you have access to healthy food and clean water in your neighborhood?"**

   Understanding Mr. Juan's access to essential resources like food and water allows the team to address nutritional deficiencies that may exacerbate his condition.

- **"Are there any recreational or exercise facilities available in your neighborhood, such as parks or gyms?"**

    This question uncovers whether Mr. Juan's living environment supports a healthy lifestyle, which is crucial in managing his overall well-being.

Next Steps for the Radiology Team: Comprehensive and Personalized Support

- Scheduling Procedure: Align with Available Transportation Options

    Flexible Scheduling: Considering Mr. Juan's remote location and transportation difficulties, the team can coordinate his CT scan around his transportation availability, including offering appointments during times when transportation services are more accessible.

- Transportation Support: Remove Barriers to Access

    Offer Transportation Assistance: The radiology team can explore transportation options through Medicaid or local non-emergency medical transport services to ensure that Mr. Juan can attend his appointments without added stress or financial burden. Providing him with these resources ensures timely diagnostic care.

- Economic Stability: Connect to Resources

    Financial Counseling and Social Support: If Mr. Juan is facing economic hardships, the radiology team should refer him to a hospital social worker who can assist in applying for financial aid, navigating healthcare costs, and accessing resources such as food and housing assistance programs.

Key Statements for Supporting Mr. Juan's Health Journey

- Transportation Support

    "We understand that transportation can be challenging for you in your rural area. Our team is here to help arrange transportation options so you can attend your medical appointments without stress. Let us know if you need assistance coordinating your travel."

- Access to Healthcare Resources

    "Given the limited healthcare services in your area, we are committed to helping you access the care you need. Please share any concerns you have about transportation, financial costs, or other barriers, and we will work together to find solutions that support your health."

- Symptoms and Health Assessment

"Your symptoms of severe coughing and shortness of breath are concerning, especially given your previous work in construction. We will conduct a thorough evaluation to determine the cause of your symptoms and provide you with the best possible care."

- Health Education on Lung Diseases

"Considering your potential exposure to asbestos and other hazardous materials during your time in construction, it is important to monitor your lung health closely. We can provide you with information on the risks associated with your occupational exposure and discuss any necessary steps for your ongoing care."

- Collaboration for Comfortable Care

"Our goal is to make your experience at the radiology department as smooth as possible. We are here to answer your questions and ensure that you feel comfortable throughout your lung CT scan process, including helping you navigate any healthcare access challenges."

Conclusion: Navigating Environmental Barriers and Accessing Care

In Mr. Juan's case, addressing the challenges posed by his neighborhood and built environment is essential to providing comprehensive care. By offering flexible scheduling, transportation support, and financial counseling, the radiology team can help him overcome barriers related to his rural location, low-income status, and potential asbestos exposure. Through patient-centered care, Mr. Juan will receive the diagnostic imaging necessary to confirm his lung condition and move forward with a treatment plan tailored to his unique needs.

Resources for Supporting Mr. Juan and Addressing SDOH Challenges

- Stanford Palo Alto Hospital Transportation Services
    - Complimentary Transportation: Free patient and visitor transportation services are available on the Stanford main hospital campus. On-demand transportation is also provided for patients with limited mobility.
    - Contact: TransportationServices@stanfordhealthcare.org
      Phone: 650.736.8000
    - More Information: Stanford Hospital Transportation

- Medi-Cal Transportation Services
  - Service Description: Medi-Cal Advantage programs offer transportation to and from doctor appointments, ensuring that patients like Mr. Juan can access necessary medical care.
  - Learn More: <u>Medi-Cal Information</u> | Phone: 855.200.7544
- National Low-Income Housing Coalition (NLIHC)
  - Support Services: The NLIHC advocates for policies that promote equitable access to affordable housing. They offer information on improving living conditions for individuals like Mr. Juan in low-income housing.
  - Explore Resources: <u>National Low-Income Housing Coalition</u>
- Asbestos.com
  - Occupational Health Support: Asbestos.com provides comprehensive resources for individuals exposed to asbestos in the workplace. They offer guidance on medical care and legal support for those affected.
  - Visit: <u>Asbestos.com</u>
- Supplemental Nutrition Assistance Program (SNAP)
  - Nutritional Assistance: SNAP offers food benefits to low-income individuals, helping them access nutritious

food and manage grocery costs, which is vital for Mr. Juan's health.
- More Information: SNAP

By addressing the social drivers of health impacting Mr. Juan's life, such as transportation barriers, economic instability, and limited access to nutritious food, the radiology team can deliver holistic care that goes beyond diagnostics. This comprehensive approach empowers patients like Mr. Juan to overcome significant challenges and take control of their health journey.

6. Case Study 6: Addressing Healthcare Access and Quality for Susan Taylor

Patient Profile: Susan Taylor Susan Taylor, a 55-year-old part-time retail worker, has a history of hypertension and diabetes. She has not had a mammogram in over five years due to financial constraints and her caregiving responsibilities for her elderly mother. Recently, she discovered a lump in her right breast during a self-examination, prompting her primary care physician (PCP) to order an urgent mammogram. Susan's situation highlights the challenges many women face in accessing preventive healthcare while managing chronic conditions and caregiving duties. The radiology team at Stanford must provide her with comprehensive support to address her unique healthcare and financial challenges.

Key Questions for the Mammography Team: Uncovering Barriers and Providing Tailored Support

To fully understand Susan's situation and provide her with the necessary care, the mammography team can ask the following questions:

- **"Do you have support to help with your mother's care while you attend your medical appointments?"**

    This will help the team determine if Susan has caregiving support or if additional resources are needed to ensure her mother's care is uninterrupted.

- **"Are there any community services that you currently use to assist with caregiving or other needs?"**

    Identifying existing support networks can help the team recommend additional resources, such as respite care or community programs, to ease her caregiving responsibilities.

- **"Do you have any concerns about scheduling or attending future medical appointments?"**

    Understanding any scheduling conflicts or transportation barriers will allow the team to provide flexible appointment options that suit Susan's needs.

- **"Do you understand the results of your mammogram and the treatment options available to you?"**

  Ensuring that Susan comprehends her diagnosis and the next steps is crucial for her peace of mind and proactive involvement in her care.

- **"Would you like additional information on managing your hypertension and diabetes alongside your cancer treatment?"**

  Offering support for her chronic conditions during cancer treatment will help Susan manage her overall health and prevent complications.

- **"Do you have any concerns about the costs associated with your treatment and follow-up care?"**

  By addressing financial concerns early, the team can connect Susan with financial counselors or Medicaid services to alleviate her stress.

Next Steps for the Mammography Team: Comprehensive Support for Susan Taylor

- Chronic Condition Management:

    Collaborate with a Dietician: Given Susan's hypertension and diabetes, the mammography team should ensure her medications are properly adjusted during her breast cancer treatment. Collaborating with a dietician can also help manage her chronic conditions with nutritional guidance that supports her overall health.

- Assistance with Paperwork:

    Help Navigating Medicaid: Understanding that Susan may be overwhelmed with financial concerns, the team can help her navigate Medicaid paperwork, ensuring that all necessary services are covered. This step can provide her with financial relief and allow her to focus on her health and recovery.

- Care Coordination:

    Assign a Nurse Navigator: A nurse navigator can guide Susan through the entire diagnostic and treatment process, from scheduling appointments to understanding her mammogram results and discussing treatment options. They can also coordinate with Susan's primary care physician to manage her chronic conditions alongside her cancer care. Additionally, the nurse navigator can provide referrals to counseling services to help Susan cope with the emotional toll of her diagnosis and caregiving responsibilities.

Key Statements for Patient-Centered Care

- Collaboration for Timely Mammogram Access:

  "We are dedicated to supporting you in accessing timely mammogram services, considering your financial and caregiving challenges. Let's work together to ensure you receive the care you need without delay."

- Comfortable and Informed Mammogram Procedure:

  "Your medical history is important to us, and we will take your hypertension and diabetes into consideration during the mammogram. We will ensure that you are comfortable and informed every step of the way."

- Patient-Centered Care and Accommodations:

  "Your comfort is our priority. Please let us know if you need any specific accommodations during your mammogram procedure so we can make your experience as smooth as possible."

Conclusion: Ensuring Holistic Care for Susan Taylor

Susan's case underscores the importance of a comprehensive approach to care that goes beyond the medical procedure itself. By addressing her financial constraints, caregiving duties, and chronic conditions, the radiology team can help her focus on her health and recovery. Providing personalized care coordination, financial assistance, and emotional support will empower Susan to manage her breast cancer diagnosis effectively while balancing her responsibilities. This case study highlights the importance of healthcare access and quality in ensuring positive health outcomes for individuals facing multiple life challenges.

Resources for Susan Taylor: Support for Healthcare Access and Financial Assistance

- Medicaid & CHIP Coverage
    - Description: Medicaid and the Children's Health Insurance Program (CHIP) provide free or low-cost health coverage to eligible individuals, including low-income families, seniors, and individuals with disabilities.
    - Website: Medicaid & CHIP Coverage Information

- Medicare - State Health Insurance Assistance Programs (SHIPs)

    o Description: Medicare provides health insurance for individuals aged 65 and older, along with certain younger individuals with disabilities. SHIPs offer personalized counseling and assistance to help beneficiaries navigate Medicare coverage.

    o Access Resources: <u>Medicare State Health Insurance Assistance Programs</u>

- COBRA (Consolidated Omnibus Budget Reconciliation Act)

    o Description: COBRA allows employees and their dependents to continue their health insurance coverage temporarily after losing employer-sponsored coverage due to a qualifying event.

    o Learn More: <u>COBRA Law Overview</u>

- Stanford Financial Counseling Services

    o Description: Stanford Health Care offers comprehensive financial counseling services to help patients navigate insurance coverage, apply for financial assistance, and manage healthcare costs effectively.

    o Contact: Palo Alto: 650.498.2900 | Tri-Valley: 925.534.6457

- o   Explore More: <u>Stanford Financial Counseling</u>
- National Breast and Cervical Cancer Early Detection Program (NBCCEDP)
    - o   Description: The NBCCEDP provides free or low-cost breast and cervical cancer screenings for eligible women who are uninsured or underinsured.
    - o   Access Information: <u>National Breast and Cervical Cancer Program</u>

By leveraging these resources and offering comprehensive support, the radiology team can help ensure that Susan receives the care and assistance she needs to successfully navigate her cancer diagnosis and treatment.

7. Case Study 7: Addressing Sex and Gender Discrimination in Healthcare

Patient Profile: Taylor Taylor, a 25-year-old individual who identifies as nonbinary and uses they/them pronouns, was assigned female at birth and is scheduled for a pelvic ultrasound examination at a radiology center. During the procedure, the sonographer unintentionally misgenders Taylor by using incorrect pronouns. When Taylor kindly corrects the sonographer, they feel a mix of discomfort and vulnerability, which intensifies their anxiety about the transvaginal ultrasound. This experience underscores the importance of creating a respectful and gender-affirming environment in healthcare, especially during sensitive medical procedures.

Key Questions for the Radiology Team: Supporting Taylor's Gender Identity and Providing Affirming Care

To ensure Taylor's comfort and respect their identity, the radiology team can ask the following questions:

- "How would you like us to address you and refer to you during your healthcare appointments?" By asking this question, the team signals respect for Taylor's identity and creates an environment where they feel seen and validated.

- "Are there specific preferences or accommodations we can provide to ensure you feel respected and comfortable during the ultrasound procedure?" This question gives Taylor the opportunity to express any particular needs, helping the team provide a more personalized and comfortable experience.

- "Is there anything you would like to share with us about your gender identity or any concerns you have about the ultrasound examination?" Encouraging Taylor to share concerns will enable the team to tailor their approach to the procedure and address any specific anxieties.

- "Can you tell us if there are any past experiences or information about your gender identity that would help us provide the best care for you today?" This question allows Taylor to share any previous healthcare experiences that may impact how they approach this ultrasound, helping the team anticipate potential discomfort.

- "How can we better support you and make this experience more affirming and positive for you?" Inviting feedback on how to improve their care reinforces the team's commitment to creating a supportive, affirming, and respectful healthcare environment.

Next Steps for the Radiology Team: Creating an Inclusive and Affirming Environment

- Comprehensive LGBTQ+ Training for Staff:

    Provide additional education on gender diversity: It is crucial for all staff members, from reception to medical technicians, to undergo continuous training on gender identity, pronoun usage, and creating affirming environments. This will help prevent situations like misgendering and ensure respectful communication at all times.

- Develop Clear Guidelines for Using Chosen Names and Pronouns:

  Implement consistent protocols: Establishing clear guidelines for consistently using patients' chosen names and pronouns in medical records, during interactions, and in all paperwork ensures that Taylor and other gender-diverse individuals are respected throughout their healthcare journey.

- Offer Gender-Affirming Educational Resources:

  Provide patient education materials that reflect diverse gender identities and specific health concerns relevant to transgender, nonbinary, and gender-diverse (TGD) individuals. Offering gender-affirming resources can reassure Taylor that the radiology team is knowledgeable about their healthcare needs.

- Tailor Support During Imaging Procedures:

  Address patient anxieties proactively: Imaging procedures can be stressful, especially for TGD individuals. The radiology team can provide additional support by allowing breaks during procedures, offering options for same-gender providers, and communicating regularly to ensure Taylor's comfort.

- Collaborate with LGBTQ+ Advocacy Groups:

    Build partnerships with LGBTQ+ organizations to improve the healthcare environment and to stay updated on best practices for supporting TGD individuals. Partnering with advocacy groups will foster a culture of inclusivity, helping healthcare providers address the unique concerns of patients like Taylor.

Key Statements for Patient-Centered, Affirming Care

- Respectful Communication Support:

    "We want to ensure that all our interactions reflect your gender identity and that you feel respected throughout your healthcare experience. Please let us know your preferred name and pronouns, and we will use them consistently during your care."

- Enhanced Comfort and Support:

    "Your comfort is our top priority. If there are any specific accommodations or adjustments that would help you feel more at ease during your ultrasound, please let us know, and we will make those arrangements."

- Affirming Environment Coordination:

    "We are committed to creating an environment where you feel safe, respected, and affirmed in your identity. Please share any concerns or preferences with us, and we will work together to ensure your care reflects your needs."

Conclusion: Ensuring Affirming and Inclusive Care for Taylor

Taylor's experience as a nonbinary individual undergoing a pelvic ultrasound highlights the importance of creating a healthcare environment that is respectful, inclusive, and affirming. Misgendering, whether unintentional or not, can significantly impact a patient's sense of safety and well-being. By asking open-ended questions about gender identity, implementing consistent practices for using chosen names and pronouns, and providing staff training on LGBTQ+ inclusivity, the radiology team can create a more positive healthcare experience for Taylor and all TGD individuals. Additionally, providing emotional support, gender-affirming care options, and addressing patient anxieties during sensitive procedures ensures a holistic approach to healthcare.

Resources for Taylor: Gender-Affirming Care and LGBTQ+ Support

- THRIVE (Therapeutic, Healing, Resilience, Inclusivity, Values, Empowerment)
    - Description: THRIVE is Stanford's LGBTQIA+ Health Program offering affirming mental health care in collaboration with primary care providers and specialists. THRIVE provides integrative, strengths-based approaches to care for individuals across the gender and sexuality spectrum.
    - Contact: 650.498.3333
    - Website: Stanford THRIVE Program

- The National Center for Transgender Equality (NCTE)
    - Description: NCTE advocates for transgender individuals' rights and provides resources for accessing gender-affirming healthcare, navigating legal issues, and connecting with local support networks.
    - Access Information: National Center for Transgender Equality

- Trans Lifeline
    - Description: Trans Lifeline provides crisis support, resources, and peer support services for transgender and gender-diverse individuals.

- Contact: 877-565-8860 (available 24/7)
- Website: Trans Lifeline

- LGBT National Help Center

  - Description: The LGBT National Help Center offers free and confidential peer support and resource information to people in need. They provide specialized hotlines for youth, seniors, and transgender individuals.
  - Access Support: LGBT National Help Center

- GLAAD Media Reference Guide

  - Description: This comprehensive guide offers best practices for respectful and accurate language use regarding LGBTQ+ identities. It is an excellent resource for healthcare providers seeking to improve their understanding of gender diversity and inclusive communication.
  - Access Guide: GLAAD Media Reference Guide

By implementing these inclusive practices and utilizing available resources, the radiology team can create a safe, respectful, and affirming space for Taylor and other LGBTQ+ patients, promoting better healthcare outcomes, and fostering a supportive healthcare environment.

Four (4) Key Takeaways

1. **Patient-Centered Care Requires Addressing Social Determinants of Health (SDOH):** Effective radiology care must incorporate a holistic approach that takes into account patients' cultural, linguistic, economic, and social barriers. Addressing these factors—such as language preferences, transportation challenges, or financial strain—ensures more equitable and compassionate care, leading to improved patient outcomes.

2. **Cultural Competency and Sensitivity Foster Trust and Improved Care:** Understanding a patient's cultural and religious background is essential for personalized care. Healthcare providers, especially in radiology, must be sensitive to gender preferences, cultural practices, and language barriers to create a comfortable environment, build trust, and provide effective care.

3. **Economic Barriers Can Limit Access to Essential Diagnostic Services:** Financial constraints, transportation issues, and work-related conflicts are significant challenges that impact patients' access to timely radiological care. Offering flexible scheduling, transportation assistance, and financial counseling helps mitigate these barriers and improve health outcomes for economically disadvantaged patients.

4. **Educational Support and Health Literacy Are Key to Patient Empowerment:** Low health literacy can lead to delays in seeking care and mismanagement of health conditions. Radiology teams must provide clear, simplified medical explanations, use visual aids, and offer language support to ensure that patients understand their diagnosis and treatment options, empowering them to take control of their health.

SECTION 4

TECHNOLOGICAL INNOVATIONS AND HEALTH EQUITY AT STANFORD MEDICINE

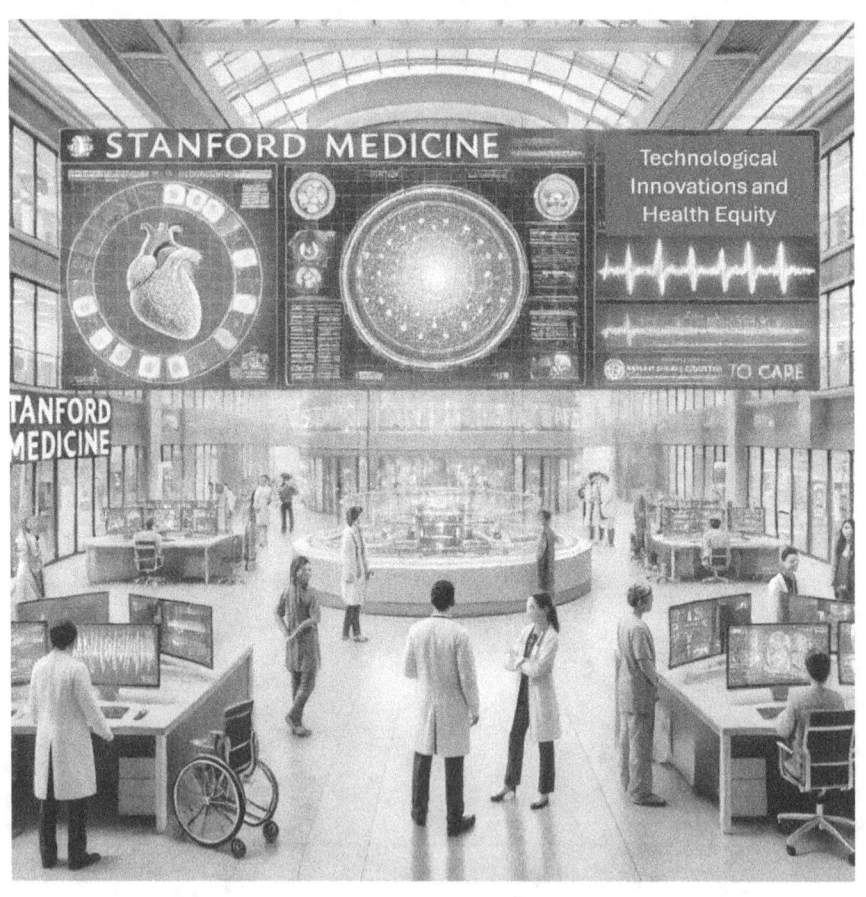

Technological Innovations and Health Equity at Stanford Medicine

Introduction

In today's rapidly evolving healthcare landscape, artificial intelligence (AI) and machine learning (ML) are emerging as transformative tools with the potential to revolutionize healthcare delivery and promote health equity. At the forefront of this revolution is Stanford Medicine, where the integration of AI into medical practices is not only enhancing diagnosis and treatment but also striving to close the gap in healthcare disparities, particularly for low-income and under-resourced populations. However, while AI holds immense promise, it also carries risks, particularly concerning the perpetuation of biases and inequalities that have long plagued marginalized communities.

AI as a Catalyst for Health Equity

The introduction of AI into healthcare has opened up possibilities for low and middle-income countries (LMICs) and underserved populations. By processing vast amounts of digital data quickly, AI enables more precise identification of diseases, facilitating earlier interventions. This can be particularly beneficial for communities with limited access to medical specialists or advanced healthcare services. AI-driven tools, such as automated note-taking during patient consultations and AI-based diagnostic tools, are freeing up time for healthcare providers, allowing them to focus on more meaningful patient interactions and address pressing health concerns, thus alleviating provider burnout.

Zuckerburg San Francisco General Hospital demonstrated how AI can address health disparities through targeted interventions. Leveraging AI, the hospital identified high-risk heart failure patients, particularly Black men with substance use disorders and housing instability, and provided them with tailored care. This case exemplifies the ability of AI to improve outcomes for vulnerable groups by directing resources where they are most needed. However, for AI to truly be a catalyst for health equity, it must be carefully implemented to avoid perpetuating the biases present in historical healthcare data.

The Risk of AI Perpetuating Bias

Despite its potential, AI's ability to exacerbate existing disparities is a legitimate concern. Several studies have revealed that AI systems can unintentionally worsen health outcomes for marginalized groups when not carefully designed or monitored. For instance, a prominent study involving a popular AI system revealed a disturbing trend: the algorithm prioritized predicting healthcare costs over identifying patients who required more intensive care. As a result, Black patients, who generally had higher healthcare needs, received the same level of care as healthier White patients. This misalignment in the algorithm's objectives is a stark reminder of the consequences when AI reflects the biases embedded in existing healthcare systems.

The integration of AI into healthcare settings, particularly radiology, poses its own challenges. Although AI training programs exist for radiologists, they are often short, sporadic, and not seamlessly integrated into the educational path of clinicians. A more comprehensive approach is needed to ensure that radiologists can confidently and effectively use AI tools while also addressing the inherent challenges and biases these tools may present. Such training must also focus on understanding the ethical implications of AI and how it can either reduce or exacerbate disparities based on race, gender, and socioeconomic status.

Stanford Medicine's Approach to AI and Health Equity

Recognizing these risks, Stanford Medicine has taken proactive steps to ensure that AI is used responsibly and equitably. The RAISE-Health Initiative, established in 2023 through a collaboration between the Stanford Institute for Human-Centered

Artificial Intelligence (HAI) and the School of Medicine, promotes the responsible use of AI in healthcare research, education, and patient care. This initiative underscores the importance of human-centered AI and its potential to transform healthcare when applied with caution and inclusivity in mind.

Additionally, the Stanford Center for Artificial Intelligence in Medicine and Imaging (AIMI) has brought together a multidisciplinary team of experts from over 20 departments to work on machine learning innovations. Their work focuses on using AI to improve diagnostic capabilities while actively addressing issues related to bias. For instance, AI was used at Stanford to repurpose chest CT scans to measure calcium levels in coronary arteries, a method that has shown to be as effective as dedicated scans. This technique is helping Cardiologist Alexander Sandhu and his team identify heart disease risk factors in patients early on, which can influence preventative care and reduce disparities in heart disease outcomes.

Principles for Ethical AI Use in Healthcare

For AI to fulfill its potential in promoting health equity, it is crucial to follow a set of guiding principles that ensure transparency, fairness, and inclusivity. These principles should include:

- Transparency in AI Algorithms: Patients and providers must understand how AI tools make decisions. This requires clear explanations of the algorithms' functions and the data that informs them.

- Diverse and Representative Data Sets: AI must be trained on data that reflects the diversity of the populations it serves. This reduces the risk of bias and ensures that the technology can be applied equitably across different racial, ethnic, and socioeconomic groups.

- Patient Privacy and Data Security: Protecting patient data is paramount. Strong privacy safeguards must be implemented to ensure that the use of AI does not compromise patient trust in the healthcare system.

- Collaboration Between Healthcare Providers and AI Developers: Ongoing collaboration between clinicians and AI developers ensures that AI tools are designed with clinical relevance in mind and are aligned with evidence-based practices.

- Regular Monitoring and Evaluation: AI systems must be regularly audited for bias and effectiveness, with adjustments made as needed to improve fairness and patient outcomes.

AI in Radiology: Balancing Innovation and Ethics

In radiology, AI's ability to process vast quantities of imaging data holds significant potential for improving diagnostic accuracy and patient care. However, AI systems must be developed with a clear focus on combating bias, particularly when dealing with racial and ethnic disparities in healthcare. Radiology departments, such as those at Stanford, are actively working to ensure that AI-driven imaging technologies do not reinforce biases or lead to unequal care. By designing anti-bias algorithms and prioritizing the ethical development of AI tools, radiology can lead the way in equitable healthcare delivery.

Pioneering AI for a More Equitable Future

Stanford Medicine's use of AI in healthcare is a model of how technological innovation can coexist with a commitment to equity and fairness. As AI continues to reshape the medical landscape, it is imperative that its deployment be guided by a strong ethical framework that prioritizes health equity. By ensuring that AI tools are designed and implemented with diversity, inclusion, and fairness in mind, Stanford and other leading institutions can harness the power of AI to reduce health disparities and improve outcomes for all patients, regardless of their race, gender, or socioeconomic status.

Resources:

Stanford Institute for Human-Centered AI (HAI): Visit HAI

Stanford Center for Artificial Intelligence in Medicine and Imaging (AIMI): Explore AIMI

AI for Health at Stanford Medicine: Learn More

Ethical AI in Healthcare Toolkit: Access the Toolkit

Four (4) Key Takeaway

1. **AI as a Tool for Advancing Health Equity:** Artificial intelligence (AI) offers transformative potential to reduce healthcare disparities, especially for underserved and low-income populations. By enabling earlier diagnosis and more precise treatments, AI can expand access to specialized care in communities with limited resources, improving overall patient outcomes.

2. **The Risk of AI Perpetuating Bias:** While AI can enhance healthcare delivery, it also carries the risk of exacerbating existing health disparities if algorithms are trained on biased data. Careful design, implementation, and continuous monitoring of AI systems are necessary to prevent reinforcing racial, gender, and socioeconomic biases in healthcare.

3. **Stanford Medicine's Responsible AI Initiatives:** Through initiatives like the RAISE-Health Initiative and AIMI, Stanford Medicine is pioneering efforts to ensure AI is developed and used ethically. These efforts emphasize transparency, fairness, and inclusivity, promoting AI tools that address healthcare disparities rather than perpetuate them.

4. **Ethical AI Development Requires Collaboration and Accountability:** The responsible use of AI in healthcare hinges on collaboration between clinicians, AI developers, and ethicists. Regular audits of AI systems, diverse datasets, and

transparent decision-making processes are critical to ensuring that AI technologies promote health equity while safeguarding patient privacy and trust.

SECTION 5

INFLUENCE OF ACADEMIC MEDICAL CENTERS IN ADVANCING HEALTH EQUITY

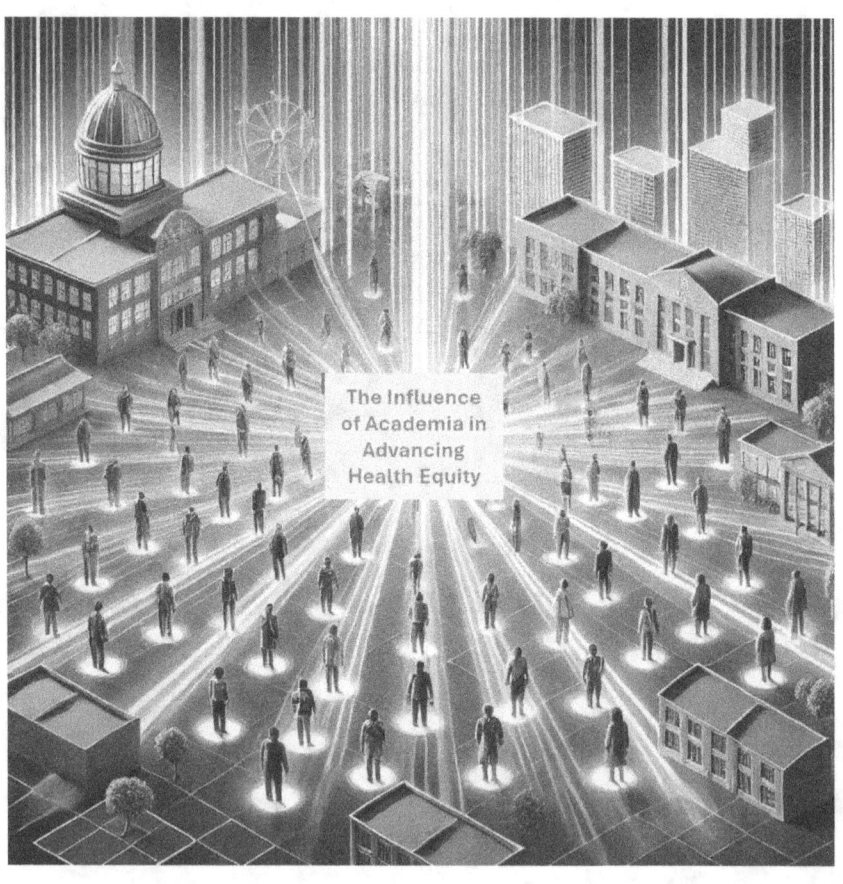

Influence of Academic Medical Centers

Introduction

Radiology departments across academic medical centers in the eastern region have embraced a pivotal role in addressing healthcare disparities and promoting health equity in local communities. By creating and implementing radiology-specific initiatives focused on community health, these institutions are not only improving patient care but also ensuring that underserved populations receive the attention and resources they need. Central to these efforts is the commitment to understanding and addressing the social drivers of health (SDOH), particularly in diverse and multilingual populations, as well as tackling critical issues exacerbated by the COVID-19 pandemic.

Radiology-Specific Initiatives and Innovations

Academic medical centers have taken significant steps in developing programs that aim to improve healthcare access for vulnerable populations. For example, many centers have launched transportation assistance programs designed to help patients with limited access to reliable transportation attend their imaging appointments. This initiative, piloted for MRI appointments, showed a marked improvement in punctuality and overall patient adherence to care plans. Elderly, unemployed, and uninsured patients especially benefited from the program, reducing no-show rates and improving diagnostic follow-ups.

Additionally, many institutions have expanded breast cancer screening services, offering extended hours and same-day mammogram options at multiple, convenient locations. This approach aims to reduce the barriers caused by busy schedules, ensuring that women—particularly those from underserved communities—do not miss out on this vital preventive measure. By addressing disparities in breast cancer detection, these initiatives directly target higher mortality rates, often found in marginalized populations due to delayed diagnosis.

Focus on Diversity, Equity, and Inclusion (DEI) in Radiology

Many academic radiology departments have secured substantial funding to support research focused on diversity, equity, and inclusion (DEI) and healthcare disparities. Training grants have been awarded to enhance the advancement of underrepresented minority groups in radiology research, and these efforts have led to numerous publications that highlight the progress made in tackling health disparities. Annual diversity weeks provide platforms for ongoing discussions around DEI, fostering collaboration among radiologists, healthcare professionals, and community leaders. These events have become key opportunities for continuing education on how radiology can be a force for health equity.

Best Practices in Addressing Health Disparities

Radiology departments are committed to implementing equitable practices that cater to the specific needs of diverse patient populations. This includes prioritizing cultural competency, sensitivity, and diversity in all aspects of care, from LGBTQ+ inclusivity to addressing the unique health needs of racial and ethnic minorities.

For example, best practices for LGBTQ+ imaging care emphasize the importance of using gender-affirming communication, respecting patient identities, ensuring privacy and confidentiality, and collaborating with LGBTQ+ communities to improve healthcare delivery. The integration of these principles in radiology helps create a welcoming environment for individuals from all backgrounds and ensures they receive the high-quality care they deserve.

Radiologists can leverage community-based participatory research (CBPR) and the NIMHD Research Framework to engage historically underserved populations. By building trust and fostering collaboration, these frameworks provide avenues for conducting impactful research that reduces access barriers and promotes health equity in imaging services.

Challenges in Promoting Health Equity

Despite the progress made, advancing health equity in radiology presents significant challenges. Women's health, particularly around maternal mortality and reproductive healthcare, remains an area where disparities persist. For rural communities, challenges related to healthcare access, such as limited access to advanced imaging technologies and shortages of healthcare professionals, continue to hinder progress. In LGBTQ+ healthcare, overcoming discrimination and improving access to gender-affirming care remain ongoing priorities.

The implementation of cultural competency programs is critical in radiology, especially in areas with diverse populations. Ensuring that radiologists and healthcare workers are equipped with the necessary skills to communicate effectively and respectfully with patients from different cultural backgrounds is essential to delivering equitable care.

Moreover, securing sustainable funding for health equity initiatives remains a challenge for many academic medical centers. While grant funding and donations have propelled initial efforts, maintaining the long-term viability of these programs will require ongoing support from both institutional leadership and government agencies.

Overcoming Disparities in Imaging Access

Addressing disparities in imaging utilization and access to advanced diagnostic technologies is vital to promoting health equity in radiology. Ensuring that all patient populations, including those in underserved communities, have access to MRI, CT scans, and other advanced imaging modalities is a top priority. Expanding the use of mobile imaging units in rural areas or offering telemedicine consultations for follow-up care can help bridge gaps in access.

Additionally, improving diversity among radiologists, technologists, and support staff is crucial. By recruiting from underrepresented groups, radiology departments can better reflect the populations they serve and foster a culturally competent workforce. Training programs must prioritize this to ensure that care is delivered with sensitivity to the unique challenges faced by patients from diverse backgrounds.

Leveraging Technology to Enhance Access

The increasing role of artificial intelligence (AI) and machine learning (ML) in radiology presents both opportunities and challenges in addressing health disparities. AI has the potential to reduce disparities by providing faster, more accurate diagnoses. However, biases in AI algorithms—if not carefully managed—can perpetuate existing inequalities in healthcare. Radiologists must work closely with AI developers to ensure that algorithms are trained on diverse data sets and that they do not reinforce biases based on race, gender, or socioeconomic status.

By leveraging technology and promoting patient-centered care, radiologists can ensure that patients are more actively involved in decision-making processes and have access to the imaging services they need, regardless of their background.

Conclusion

The Stanford Health Care (SHC) Radiology Resource on Social Drivers of Health (SDOH) and Advancing Health Equity is designed to support radiology departments and healthcare professionals in their efforts to promote health equity, improve patient outcomes, and reduce the cost of care. By following the best practices outlined in this guide, radiology professionals can continue to advance the cause of inclusive, patient-centered care that addresses health disparities head-on.

Moving forward, academic medical centers must remain committed to fostering diversity and equity within their departments, conducting impactful research, and continuously monitoring the progress of health equity initiatives. Collaboration across medical specialties, community partnerships, and ongoing staff training will be essential to ensuring that radiology departments.

Four (4) Key Takeaway

1. **Radiology-Specific Initiatives for Improved Access:** Academic medical centers are leading efforts to promote health equity by developing programs like transportation assistance for underserved populations and expanding breast cancer screening services. These initiatives have been instrumental in reducing barriers to care, improving punctuality for imaging appointments, and increasing access to vital diagnostic services for marginalized communities.

2. **Diversity, Equity, and Inclusion (DEI) in Radiology:** Academic radiology departments are securing funding and advancing research focused on healthcare disparities and DEI. Through diversity weeks, training grants, and publications, they are driving awareness and education around the unique needs of underrepresented populations, fostering a culture of inclusivity and collaboration in radiology.

3. **Addressing Health Disparities through Best Practices:** Radiology departments are implementing culturally competent and inclusive practices, such as gender-affirming care and community-based participatory research (CBPR), to ensure equitable care delivery. These efforts focus on engaging underserved populations, improving access to imaging, and reducing disparities based on race, gender, and socioeconomic status.

4. **Leveraging Technology for Equity in Radiology:** The integration of AI and mobile imaging units is helping to bridge gaps in access to advanced diagnostic technologies. However, the ethical use of AI requires careful management to avoid perpetuating biases. Radiology departments must work closely with AI developers to ensure equitable, bias-free technological solutions that enhance healthcare access for all populations.

REFERENCES

"About SDOH in Healthcare." *Www.ahrq.gov*, www.ahrq.gov/sdoh/about.html#:~:text=These%20can%20include%3A. Accessed 30 July 2024.

accfb. "Get Food Today from Alameda County Community Food Bank." *Alameda County Community Food Bank*, www.accfb.org/get-food. Accessed 30 July 2024.

Affairs, img src='/content/sm-profiles/tracie_white/_jcr_content/image img 620 high jpg/profileTWhiteM jpg' alt='Tracie White'> Tracie White Tracie White is a science writer for the medical school's Office of Communication & Public. "Lesbian, Gay, Bisexual and Transgendered Health Issues Not Being Taught at Medical Schools, Study Finds." *News Center*, 10 Mar. 2009, med.stanford.edu/news/all-news/2011/09/lesbian-gay-bisexual-and-transgendered-health-issues-not-being-taught-at-medical-schools-study-finds.html. Accessed 30 July 2024.

Armitage, Hanae. "Researchers Create Guide for Fair and Equitable AI in Health Care." *Scope*, 3 Oct. 2022, scopeblog.stanford.edu/2022/10/03/researchers-create-guide-for-fair-and-equitable-ai-in-healthcare/.

Arthur, Sophie, et al. "Medical Students' Awareness of Health Issues, Attitudes, and Confidence about Caring for Lesbian,

Gay, Bisexual and Transgender Patients: A Cross-Sectional Survey." *BMC Medical Education*, vol. 21, no. 1, 14 Jan. 2021, bmcmededuc.biomedcentral.com/articles/10.1186/s12909-020-02409-6, https://doi.org/10.1186/s12909-020-02409-6.

Avalos, George, and The Mercury News. "Tech Job Cuts Ease a Bit in Bay Area as Industry Layoffs Haunt Region." *Techxplore.com*, techxplore.com/news/2024-05-tech-job-ease-bit-bay.html. Accessed 30 July 2024.

Bavli, Itai, and David S. Jones. "Race Correction and the X-Ray Machine — the Controversy over Increased Radiation Doses for Black Americans in 1968." *New England Journal of Medicine*, vol. 387, no. 10, 8 Sept. 2022, pp. 947–952, https://doi.org/10.1056/nejmms2206281.

Bennett, John. "ClinicalKey." *Clinicalkey.com*, Elsevier, 2020, www.clinicalkey.com/#.

Bohn, Sarah, et al. "Poverty in California - Public Policy Institute of California." Public Policy Institute of California, 2019, www.ppic.org/publication/poverty-in-california/.

Boyd-Barrett, Claudia. "Is AI Good for Health Equity? California Leaders Weigh In." *California Health Care Foundation*, 9 May 2024, www.chcf.org/blog/is-ai-good-health-equity-california-leaders-weigh-in/#:~:text=But%20the%20prodigious%20power%20of. Accessed 30 July 2024.

"Community Partnerships." *Stanfordhealthcare.org*, stanfordhealthcare.org/about-us/community-partnerships.html.

Conley, Mark. "How Stanford Medicine Is Capturing the AI Moment." *Stanford Medicine Magazine*, 10 Nov. 2023, stanmed.stanford.edu/translating-ai-concepts-into-innovations/.

Cull • •, Ian. "Census Data Shows How the Bay Area Changed over the Last 10 Years." *NBC Bay Area*, 26 May 2023, www.nbcbayarea.com/news/local/census-bay-area-population/3238075/. Accessed 30 July 2024.

DeBenedectis, Carolynn M., et al. "Health Care Disparities in Radiology—a Review of the Current Literature." *Journal of the American College of Radiology*, vol. 19, no. 1, Part B, 1 Jan. 2022, pp. 101–111, www.sciencedirect.com/science/article/pii/S1546144021007432, https://doi.org/10.1016/j.jacr.2021.08.024.

Duggan, Tara. "The Bay Area's Hidden Problem: Hunger and Food Insecurity." *San Francisco Chronicle*, 18 Nov. 2018, www.sfchronicle.com/food/article/The-hidden-hungryA-Bay-Area-paradox-13379274.php.

Goldberg, Julia E., et al. "How We Got Here: The Legacy of Anti-Black Discrimination in Radiology." *RadioGraphics*, vol. 43, no. 2, 1 Feb. 2023, https://doi.org/10.1148/rg.220112.

Hafeez, Hudaisa, et al. "Health Care Disparities among Lesbian, Gay, Bisexual, and Transgender Youth: A Literature Review." *Cureus*, vol. 9, no. 4, 20 Apr. 2018, www.ncbi.nlm.nih.gov/pmc/articles/PMC5478215/, https://doi.org/10.7759/cureus.1184.

Haygood, Tamara Miner. "Patient Literacy and Access to Radiology Information." *Radiology*, vol. 291, no. 1, Apr. 2019, pp. 119–120, https://doi.org/10.1148/radiol.2019190007.

"Health Disparities Program | San Francisco." *Www.sf.gov*, www.sf.gov/data/health-disparities-program. Accessed 30 July 2024.

"Health Equity." *Diversity at Stanford Medicine*, med.stanford.edu/diversity/health-equity.html. Accessed 30 July 2024.

"Health Equity Resources." *Www.radhealthequity.org*, www.radhealthequity.org/Resources?topics=Social-Economic. Accessed 30 July 2024.

"Health Literacy." *HPSM*, www.hpsm.org/provider/resources/cultural-competency/health-literacy. Accessed 30 July 2024.

"Help the Food Bank Provide Meals." *Food Bank of Contra Costa and Solano*, www.foodbankccs.org.

"Hospitals and Health Equity: Examples of Novel Strategies." *OncLive*, www.chiefhealthcareexecutive.com/view/hospitals-and-health-equity-examples-of-novel-strategies.

Iv Kyrazis, Crysta B., et al. "Imaging Care for Transgender and Gender Diverse Patients: Best Practices and Recommendations." *RadioGraphics*, vol. 43, no. 2, 1 Feb. 2023, https://doi.org/10.1148/rg.220124.

Lawson, Marissa B, et al. "Comparative Performance of Contrast-Enhanced Mammography, Abbreviated Breast MRI, and Standard Breast MRI for Breast Cancer Screening." *Radiology*, vol. 308, no. 2, 1 Aug. 2023, https://doi.org/10.1148/radiol.230576.

"LGBTQ+ Health Program | Stanford Health Care." *Stanfordhealthcare.org*, stanfordhealthcare.org/medical-clinics/lgbtq-health.html.

Liu, David Shalom, et al. "Changes in Radiology due to Artificial Intelligence That Can Attract Medical Students to the Specialty." *JMIR Medical Education*, vol. 9, 20 Mar. 2023, p. e43415, https://doi.org/10.2196/43415.

Nikki Lopez Suarez, et al. "Practical Approaches to Advancing Health Equity in Radiology, from the *AJR* Special Series on DEI." *American Journal of Roentgenology*, vol. 221, no. 1, 1 July 2023, pp. 1–10, https://doi.org/10.2214/ajr.22.28783. Accessed 31 Aug. 2023.

Nine-County San Francisco Bay Area Region.

Obedin-Maliver, Juno, et al. "Lesbian, Gay, Bisexual, and Transgender–Related Content in Undergraduate Medical Education." *JAMA*, vol. 306, no. 9, 7 Sept. 2011, jamanetwork.com/journals/jama/fullarticle/1104294, https://doi.org/10.1001/jama.2011.1255.

"Race/Ethnicity | Bay Area Equity Atlas." *Bayareaequityatlas.org*, bayareaequityatlas.org/indicators/race-ethnicity.

Reid, Carolina, et al. *Housing + Climate Policy: Building Equitable Pathways to Sustainability and Affordability.*

Safdar, Nabile M. "An Introduction to Health Disparities for the Practicing Radiologist." *Journal of the American College of Radiology*, vol. 16, no. 4, Apr. 2019, pp. 542–546, https://doi.org/10.1016/j.jacr.2018.12.023.

San Francisco Bay Area Region Report CLIMATE CHANGE ASSESSMENT Introduction to California's Fourth Climate Change Assessment.

San Francisco Community Health Needs Assessment. 2019.

Sowinski, John S., and Richard B. Gunderman. "Transgender Patients: What Radiologists Need to Know." *American Journal of Roentgenology*, vol. 210, no. 5, May 2018, pp. 1106–1110, https://doi.org/10.2214/ajr.17.18904.

Stowell, Justin T., et al. "Multidisciplinary Approach to Imaging for Gender-Affirming Surgery: Engaging Surgeons, Radiologists, and Patients to Ensure a Positive Imaging Experience." *Annals of Translational Medicine*, vol. 9, no. 7, Apr. 2021, pp. 610–610, https://doi.org/10.21037/atm-20-6431.

"The Bay Area Atlas: A Data and Analysis Tool | PolicyLink." *Www.policylink.org*, www.policylink.org/our-work/economy/baea. Accessed 30 July 2024.

"The Bay Area Today | Plan Bay Area 2040 Final Plan." *2040.Planbayarea.org*, 2040.planbayarea.org/the-bay-area-today.

"THRIVE (Therapeutic, Healing, Resilience, Inclusivity, Values, Empowerment) Clinic." *Department of Psychiatry and Behavioral Sciences*, med.stanford.edu/psychiatry/patient_care/thrive.html. Accessed 30 July 2024.

"Uninsured and Unprotected: Data Shows Growing Health Insurance Gap across the Bay Area." *ABC7 San Francisco*, 29 Sept. 2021, abc7news.com/health-insurance-uninsured-hispanics-in-bay-area-gap-inequities/11045248/#:~:text=Out%20of%20all%20nine%20Bay.

Waite, Stephen, et al. "Narrowing the Gap: Imaging Disparities in Radiology." *Radiology*, vol. 299, no. 1, 9 Feb. 2021, p. 203742, https://doi.org/10.1148/radiol.2021203742.

Wandy, T, et al. "Improving Awareness of LGBTQ Patient Preferences among Radiology Staff Members." *Current Problems in Diagnostic Radiology*, Mar. 2021, https://doi.org/10.1067/j.cpradiol.2021.03.011. Accessed 20 Mar. 2021.

www.ingramcontent.com/pod-product-compliance
Lightning Source LLC
Chambersburg PA
CBHW052259220526
45471CB00001B/405